EDITORS

Imad F. Btaiche, PharmD, BCNSP
Clinical Associate Professor
University of Michigan College of Pharmacy
Clinical Pharmacist, Surgery and Nutrition Support
Program Director, Critical Care Pharmacy Residency
Department of Pharmacy Services
University of Michigan Hospitals and Health Centers

Nabil Khalidi, PharmD, FASHP
Clinical Associate Professor
Director of International Programs
University of Michigan College of Pharmacy

Debra S. Kovacevich, RN, MPH
Adjunct Clinical Assistant Professor
University of Michigan College of Pharmacy
Nurse Manager, Michigan Home Care Services, HomeMed
University of Michigan Hospitals and Health Centers

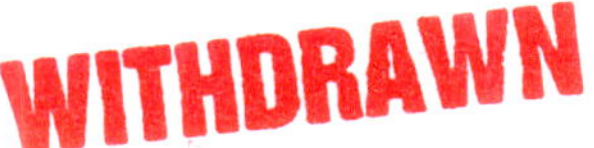

Endorsed by the Pharmacy and Therapeutics Committee with the approval of the Executive Committee on Clinical Affairs, 2009.

The printing of this manual was made possible by a grant from Hospira, Inc., Lake Forest, Illinois.

CONTRIBUTORS

Sandra F. Bouma, MS, RD
Senior Dietitian, Pediatric Bone Marrow Transplant
Patient Food and Nutrition Services
University of Michigan Hospitals and Health Centers

Imad F. Btaiche, PharmD, BCNSP
Clinical Associate Professor
University of Michigan College of Pharmacy
Clinical Pharmacist, Surgery and Nutrition Support
Program Director, Critical Care Pharmacy Residency
Department of Pharmacy Services
University of Michigan Hospitals and Health Centers

Mary Petrea Cober, BS, PharmD, BCNSP
Clinical Assistant Professor
University of Michigan College of Pharmacy
Clinical Pharmacist, Pediatric Surgery
Department of Pharmacy Services
University of Michigan Hospitals and Health Centers

Lori McCord Jordan, RD
Senior Dietitian, Trauma and Burn
Patient Food and Nutrition Services
University of Michigan Hospitals and Health Centers

Nabil Khalidi, PharmD, FASHP
Clinical Associate Professor
Director of International Programs
University of Michigan College of Pharmacy

Debra S. Kovacevich, RN, MPH
Adjunct Clinical Assistant Professor
University of Michigan College of Pharmacy
Nurse Manager, Michigan Home Care Services, HomeMed
University of Michigan Hospitals and Health Centers

Deborah A. Pasko, PharmD
Adjunct Clinical Associate Professor
University of Michigan College of Pharmacy
Clinical Pharmacist, Pediatric Intensive Care
Clinical Coordinator, Department of Pharmacy Services
University of Michigan Hospitals and Health Centers

Melissa Pleva, PharmD, BCPS, BCNSP
Adjunct Clinical Instructor
University of Michigan College of Pharmacy
Clinical Pharmacist, Surgery Critical Care and Nutrition Support
Department of Pharmacy Services
University of Michigan Hospitals and Health Centers

Jennifer A. Wooley, MS, RD, CNSD
Manager, Nutrition Services
Patient Food and Nutrition Services
University of Michigan Hospitals and Health Centers

REVIEWERS

Pamela I. Brown, MD, PhD
Associate Professor of Pediatrics and Communicable Diseases
University of Michigan Medical School
Pediatric Gastroenterology
University of Michigan Hospitals and Health Centers

Daryl D. DePestel, PharmD, BCPS
Clinical Associate Professor
University of Michigan College of Pharmacy
Clinical Pharmacist, Infectious Diseases
Department of Pharmacy Services
University of Michigan Hospitals and Health Centers

Michelle M. Johnson, RD, CSP
Senior Dietitian, Neonatal Intensive Care Unit
Patient Food and Nutrition Services
University of Michigan Hospitals and Health Centers

Michael D. Kraft, PharmD, BCNSP
Clinical Associate Professor
University of Michigan College of Pharmacy
Clinical Pharmacist, Surgery and Nutrition Support
Clinical Coordinator, Department of Pharmacy Services
University of Michigan Hospitals and Health Centers

Lena M. Napolitano, MD, FACS, FCCM, FCCP
Professor of Surgery
University of Michigan Medical School
Division Chief, Acute Care Surgery
Director, Surgical Critical Care
General Surgery
University of Michigan Hospitals and Health Centers

Sandhya Padiyar, MS, RD, CSP
Senior Dietitian, Neonatal Intensive Care Unit
Patient Food and Nutrition Services
University of Michigan Hospitals and Health Centers

Deborah A. Pasko, PharmD
Adjunct Clinical Associate Professor
University of Michigan College of Pharmacy
Clinical Pharmacist, Pediatric Intensive Care
Clinical Coordinator, Department of Pharmacy Services
University of Michigan Hospitals and Health Centers

Melissa Pleva, PharmD, BCPS, BCNSP
Adjunct Clinical Instructor
University of Michigan College of Pharmacy
Clinical Pharmacist, Surgery Critical Care and Nutrition Support
Department of Pharmacy Services
University of Michigan Hospitals and Health Centers

Robert E. Schumacher, MD
Associate Professor of Pediatrics and Communicable Diseases
University of Michigan Medical School
Neonatal-Perinatal Medicine
University of Michigan Hospitals and Health Centers

Daniel H. Teitelbaum, MD
Professor of Surgery
University of Michigan Medical School
Pediatric Surgery
University of Michigan Hospitals and Health Centers

Danielle K. Turgeon, MD
Associate Professor of Internal Medicine
University of Michigan Medical School
Gastroenterology
University of Michigan Hospitals and Health Centers

Laraine L. Washer, MD
Clinical Instructor of Internal Medicine
University of Michigan Medical School
Infectious Diseases
University of Michigan Hospitals and Health Centers

Jennifer A. Wooley, MS, RD, CNSD
Manager, Nutrition Services
Patient Food and Nutrition Services
University of Michigan Hospitals and Health Centers

ACKNOWLEDGMENTS

The editors of the Parenteral and Enteral Nutrition (PEN) Manual acknowledge the extraordinary contributions of everyone who has been involved in writing, reviewing, and in editing this manual over the past thirty years. These individuals are:

John R. Wesley, MD; Anita B. Clavier, RN; Patricia A. Saran, RN; Paul Conlon, PharmD; Nabil Khalidi, PharmD; Walter C. Faubion, RN; Wendy Baker, RN; Beth Perlmutter, RN; Susan M. Hickish, RD; Josephine M. Hogan, RN; Debra S. Kovacevich, RN; Gilbert B. Olson, PharmD; Robert A. Wolk, PharmD; Carol L. Braunschweig, RD; Christopher J. Maksym, PharmD; Cindy A. Smith, RN; Susan M. Revesz, RN; Anne M. Perez, RN; Linda A. Hager, RD; Debra Wilson, RD; Bessie Marikis, PharmD; Carol Graham, RN; Patricia C. Sirois, PharmD; Jorge L. Rodriguez, MD; Theresa L. Han-Markey, RD; Deborah Lown, RD; M. Luisa Partipilo, PharmD; Bonnie L. Peters, RN; Anthony Boney, RN; David A. August, MD; Imad F. Btaiche, PharmD; Daniel H. Teitelbaum, MD; Heather A. Rowe, RD; Michael D. Kraft, PharmD; Timothy T. Nostrant, MD; Mary H. O'Leary, RD; Robert H. Bartlett, MD; Carol E. Chenoweth, MD; Deborah M. Yonkoski, RD; Kristen A. VanDerElzen, MPH.

A special tribute is paid to the health and nutrition experts who contributed to this edition with updated concepts and procedures, and to the reviewers who kept all of us honest and on track. Without their input and insightful contributions, there would not have been a PEN manual. We also appreciate the support of Hospira, Inc. for printing this edition and Abbott Laboratories for printing all previous editions of the PEN Manual. We will be forever grateful for everybody's assistance, suggestions, and contributions.

PREFACE

The Department of Pharmacy Services at the University of Michigan, the authors, and the reviewers of this ninth edition of the Parenteral and Enteral Nutrition Manual are proud to introduce this newly revised, practical reference for clinicians who provide parenteral and enteral nutrition therapy to hospitalized and home patients. By doing so, the Department of Pharmacy Services and the parenteral and enteral nutrition clinicians at the University of Michigan Hospitals and Health Centers are upholding a thirty-year-old tradition that has resulted in publishing nine editions of this manual.

This manual, in its newest edition, provides an up-to-date practical approach to the provision of rational, effective, and safe nutrition support therapy, as practiced at the University of Michigan. It emphasizes the role of enteral nutrition and outlines the fastest and safest means for transitioning patients from parenteral to enteral nutrition, and then to oral intake. We consolidated and expanded the chapters on complications associated with parenteral and enteral nutrition and their respective management. In addition, we updated the appendix on medication compatibility with parenteral nutrition, along with the appendix on oral dosage forms that should not be crushed for administration with enteral nutrition. We also updated our guidelines to reflect the most recent critical care guidelines for nutrition support practice by the American Society for Parenteral and Enteral Nutrition (A.S.P.E.N.) and the Society for Critical Care Medicine (SCCM). Lastly, we expanded the bibliography and the index, and increased the number of interdisciplinary health professional reviewers for this edition. We are confident that clinicians and educators in the field of nutrition support will appreciate the information presented in this manual.

The Editors

ORGANIZATIONAL CHART

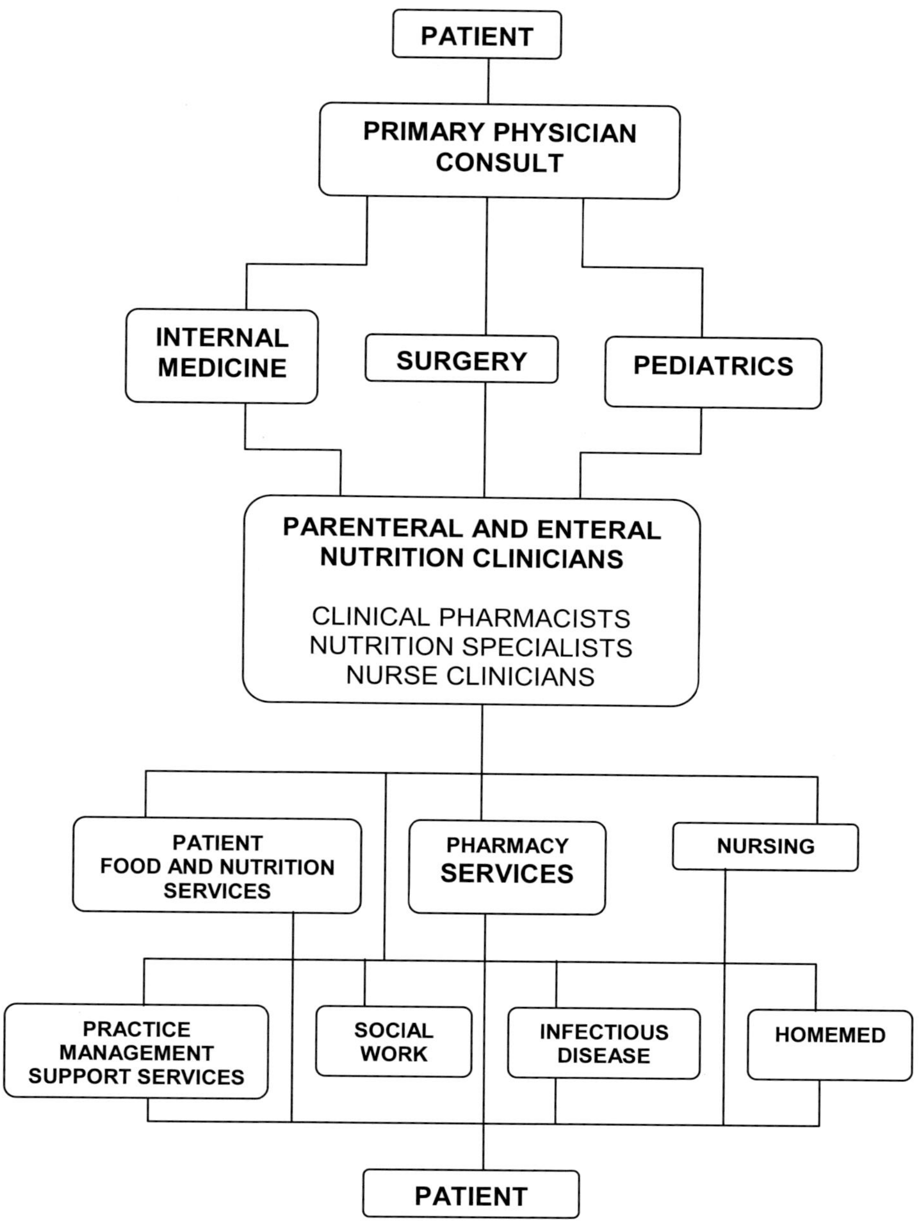

TABLE OF CONTENTS

I. INTRODUCTION

Providing optimal nutrition support therapy requires the convergence of many skills and aspects of patient care, including:

- Assessing the patient's nutritional status and nutritional requirements.
- Identifying the proper route and techniques for nutrition support therapy.
- Relating the pathophysiology of the patient's diseases; clinical conditions; diagnostic tests; laboratory parameters; medication therapy; and the nutritional, fluids, electrolytes, and acid-base balance.
- Knowing the patient's medication therapy and evaluating any possible medication-nutrient interactions.
- Appropriately formulate, administer, monitor, and adjust nutrition support therapy.

NUTRITION SUPPORT THERAPY

Nutrition support therapy refers to the provision of nutrients by the oral, enteral, or parenteral route for therapeutic reasons. Nutrition support therapy may include parenteral nutrition, enteral nutrition, and therapeutic nutrients intended to maintain or restore nutritional status and health.

PARENTERAL NUTRITION

Parenteral (PN) describes the intravenous administration of mixed fluids, amino acids, dextrose, lipid emulsions, multivitamins, trace elements, and electrolytes for the purpose of weight maintenance or gain, to preserve or restore lean body mass, to support anabolism and nitrogen balance, and to correct nutritional deficiencies in patients requiring nutrition support therapy when the oral and enteral feeding routes are inadequate, not feasible, or contraindicated.

ENTERAL NUTRITION

Enteral nutrition (EN) describes the delivery of nutrients through a tube into the gastrointestinal tract. When nutrition support therapy is indicated, EN should be used in preference to PN in patients who cannot eat and with a functional and accessible gastrointestinal tract.

II. INDICATIONS AND ROUTES OF NUTRITION SUPPORT THERAPY

Nutrition support therapy (i.e., enteral or parenteral nutrition, nutritional supplements) is not indicated in well-nourished adult patients who are under little or no metabolic stress for the first 5 to 7 days of hospitalization.

In patients who are malnourished or under metabolic stress, enteral nutrition (EN) is indicated as a first-line nutrition support therapy when the gastrointestinal tract is functional and when protein and energy needs cannot be met via the oral route. Early EN, which is initiated within 24 to 48 hours of patient admission to the intensive care unit, has shown to improve the outcomes of critically ill patients.

In well-nourished adult patients, parenteral nutrition (PN) is indicated when EN or oral nutrition is not possible, only after 5 to 7 days of hospitalization and if PN therapy is expected to last for at least 7 days. PN that is used for less than 7 days is unlikely to be of clinical benefit and may increase the risks of infectious and metabolic complications. Supplemental PN is not indicated during the first 7 to 10 days of EN, is unlikely to produce clinical benefits, and may increase the risks of complications.

In malnourished patients, PN should be started as soon as possible when EN is not feasible. In malnourished adult patients who are scheduled to undergo a major upper gastrointestinal surgery and for whom EN is not feasible, PN should be initiated 5 to 7 days pre-operatively and continued during the post-operative period until oral or EN becomes feasible.

An adult patient who meets the criteria for PN therapy would benefit from a central PN that is infused via a central venous access device, in order to provide adequate proteins and calories to meet the patient's nutritional requirements. Because limited amounts of proteins and calories can be provided in peripheral parenteral nutrition (PPN) admixtures due to solution osmolarity limitations, PPN is not expected to meet the patient's total protein and energy requirements. Further, PPN admixtures are hyperosmolar solutions that are infused into a peripheral vein, which may increase the risk of phlebitis. Therefore, PPN is not recommended particularly in adult patients. At the University of Michigan Hospitals and Health Centers, the use of PPN is restricted to adult patients (body weight > 30 kg) who are PN-dependent and who lose central venous access and will not likely be able to obtain central venous access for at least 5 to 7 days.

ROUTES TO DELIVER NUTRITION SUPPORT TO ADULTS: CLINICAL DECISION ALGORITHM

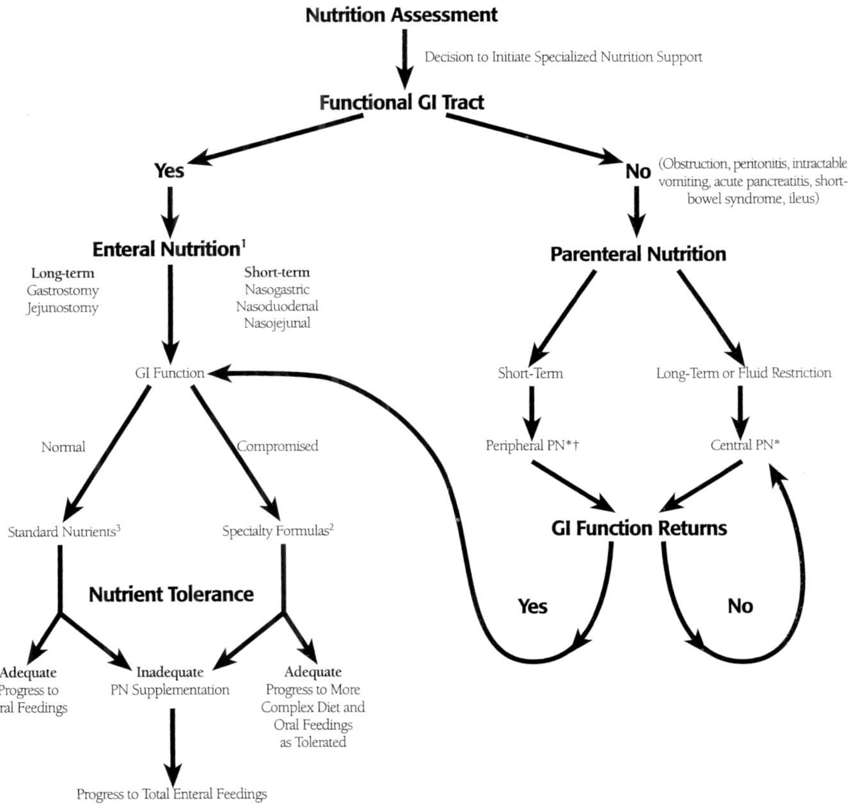

Reprinted from: A.S.P.E.N. Board of Directors. Clinical Pathways and Algorithms for Delivery of Parenteral and Enteral Nutrition Support in Adults. Silver Spring, MD: A.S.P.E.N.;1998:5; with permission from the American Society for Parenteral and Enteral Nutrition (A.S.P.E.N.). A.S.P.E.N. does not endorse the use of this material in any other form than its entirety.

Note: it is our clinical judgment that the benefits of peripheral PN (PPN) on improving patient outcomes have not been clearly demonstrated or documented

III. NUTRITION ASSESSMENT FOR ADULT PATIENTS

Nutrition assessment should be completed prior to implementing enteral nutrition (EN) or parenteral nutrition (PN). The primary goals of nutrition assessment are to identify, prevent, and correct malnutrition before it becomes a factor leading to patient morbidity or mortality. Although severely malnourished patients can be easily recognized by their physical features of wasting, patients who are moderately malnourished or with subtle nutrient deficiencies may go unnoticed and pose a diagnostic challenge. Early identification of patients with, or at risk for malnutrition constitutes the first step to provide proper nutrition support therapy. Institutional mechanisms and policies have been developed to trigger a nutrition consult and assessment by a registered dietitian for hospitalized patients. The details and policies regarding patient screening and patient referral to a registered dietitian are available from the Patient Food and Nutrition Services, "Nutrition Care Process: Screening, Assessment & Reassessment."

ASSESMENT OF NUTRITIONAL STATUS

The assessment of nutritional status incorporates subjective and objective data including a review of the medical and surgical history, diet history, anthropometric measurements, biochemical assessment, and physical evaluation as shown in Table 1.

Diet History

A detailed diet history is essential in the evaluation of nutritional status. Nutrition history requires an accurate diet history, assessment of baseline status, and detection of any subclinical nutritional deficiencies. Changes in taste, appetite, intake, weight, or consumption of special or restricted diet may suggest an altered nutritional state. Dentition, level of independence, social, religious and cultural preferences, psychosocial issues, food frequency, activity level, intake of nutrition supplements, and level of nutritional education should also be assessed. Patients with gastrointestinal resections may be at risk for malabsorption and nutritional deficiencies. Knowing the affected gastrointestinal sites where specific nutrients are absorbed is important in order to provide adequate nutrient supplementation via the appropriate route (Figure 1).

Figure 1. Intestinal Sites of Nutrients Absorption

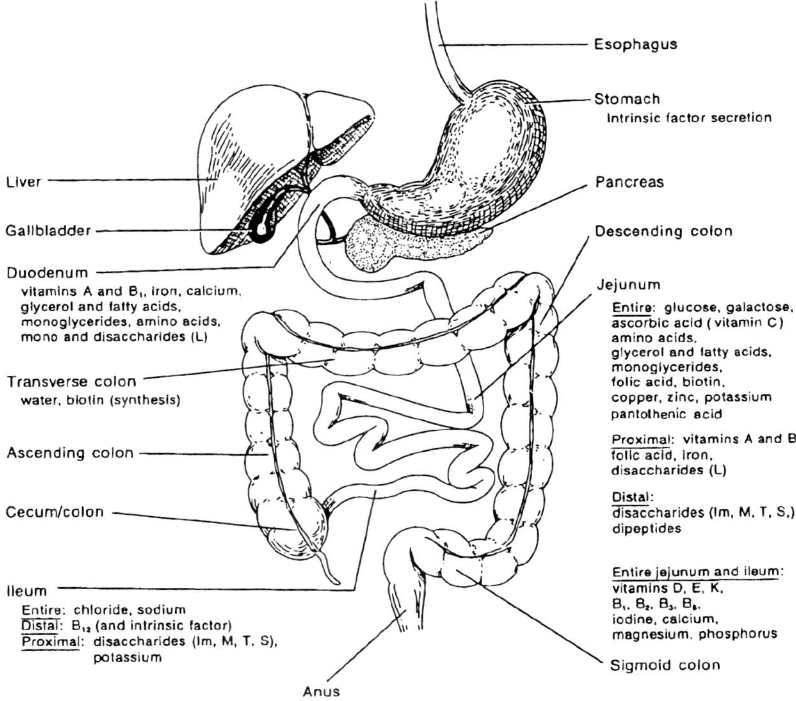

The exact sites for absorption of chromium, manganese, selenium, cadmium, cobalt, and molybdenum are unknown.
L = lactose; IM = isomaltase; M = maltase; T = trehalose; S = sucrose.
Reprinted with permission from: Caldwell MD, Kennedy-Caldwell C. Normal nutritional requirements. Surg Clin North Am 1981;61:489-507.

Anthropometric Measurements

Normal body weight or obesity does not necessarily reflect adequate nutritional status. Body weight and height are the most frequently used anthropometric measurements. Body mass index (BMI), which is calculated by dividing the body weight (kg) by the height (m^2), is a vague indicator of body fat mass in adults. Body weight status is classified based on BMI as: underweight less than 18.5; normal 18.5 to 24.9; overweight 25 to 29.9; obese 30 and over. Although not commonly used due to their inherent limitations, skinfold thickness measurements (triceps, biceps, subscapular) have been used to estimate body fat, and midarm muscle circumference as an indicator of muscle mass. Abdominal adiposity and its health-risk potential have been gaining more attention, and measurement guidelines have been proposed for appropriate waist circumference and waist-to-hip ratio. When estimating energy and protein requirements, lost body parts should be taken into consideration (Figure 2).

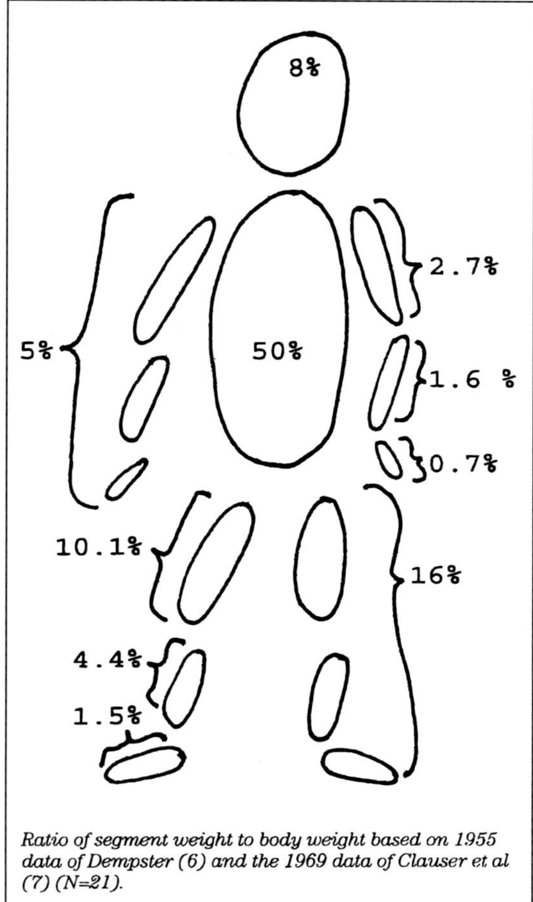

Ratio of segment weight to body weight based on 1955 data of Dempster (6) and the 1969 data of Clauser et al (7) (N=21).

Reprinted with permission from: Osterkamp LK. Current perspective on assessment of human body proportions of relevance to amputees. J Am Diet Assoc 1995;95:215-8.

Biochemical Assessment

Laboratory data include essential markers used in the assessment of nutritional status. Serum visceral proteins (e.g., prealbumin, albumin) are commonly used to assess nutritional status and response to nutrition support therapy. However, serum visceral protein concentrations may lack sensitivity and specificity as nutritional markers during severe stress and inflammation. Nitrogen balance studies can be performed to evaluate the adequacy of protein retention, and protein and caloric intake. Serum concentrations and markers of trace element, minerals, and vitamins are also measured as needed (Chapter VII).

CLASSIFICATION OF NUTRITIONAL STATUS

Acute malnutrition describes the status of a protein-depleted patient with adequate fat reserves. A hospitalized patient with acute malnutrition might be obese but under catabolic stress. Chronic malnutrition represents depletion of protein and fat stores, with the classic emaciated-appearing malnourished patient. A patient with chronic malnutrition generally has a long history of poor nutritional intake. Most hospitalized patients are somewhere between the two extremes. Several methods can be used for the assessment and classification of the patient's nutritional status. One of the methods is the subjective global assessment (SGA) described, as follows:

Normally nourished: no weight loss or recent weight loss of 0.5 to 1 kg or less (disregard if patient is edematous or has ascites), and/or no abnormal dietary intake, and/or no history or less than 2 days history of anorexia, nausea, vomiting, or diarrhea.

Moderately malnourished: weight loss of 5% to 10% of usual body weight in the past 6 months (disregard if patient is edematous or has ascites), and/or abnormal dietary intake for 1 month, and/or history of anorexia, nausea, vomiting, or diarrhea for short time.

Severely malnourished: weight loss of more than 10% of usual body weight in less than 6 months (disregard if patient has edema), and/or BMI less than 18.5, and/or inadequate dietary intake for more than 1 month, and/or history of anorexia, nausea, vomiting, or diarrhea for over 1 month, and/or visual somatic protein wasting.

Table 1. Clinical Findings on Physical Examination Related to Nutritional Alterations

Clinical findings	Consider deficiency of	Consider excess	Frequency
Hair, nails			
• Flag sign (transverse depigmentation of hair)	Protein (protein deficiency signifies Kwashiorkor)		Rare
• Easily pluckable hair	Protein		Common
• Sparse hair	Protein, biotin, zinc	Vitamin A	Occasional
• Corkscrew, unmerged coiled hair	Vitamin C		Common
• Transverse ridging of nails	Protein		Occasional
Skin			
• Scaling	Vitamin A, zinc, essential fatty acids	Vitamin A	Occasional
• Cellophane appearance	Protein		Occasional
• Cracking (flaky paint or crazy pavement dermatosis)	Protein		Rare
• Follicular hyperkeratosis	Vitamins A, C		Occasional
• Petechiae (perifollicular)	Vitamin C		Occasional
• Purpura	Vitamins C, K		Common
• Pigmentation, desquamation of sun-exposed areas	Niacin		Rare
• Yellow pigmentation-sparing sclerae (benign)		Carotene	Common
Eyes			
• Papilledema		Vitamin A	Rare
• Night blindness	Vitamin A		Rare
Perioral			
• Angular stomatitis	Riboflavin, pyridoxine, niacin		Occasional
• Cheilosis (dry, cracking, ulcerated lips)	Riboflavin, pyridoxine, niacin		Rare
Oral			
• Atrophic lingual papillae (slick tongue)	Riboflavin, niacin, folate, vitamin B12, protein, iron		Common
• Glossitis (scarlet, raw tongue)	Riboflavin, niacin, pyridoxine, folate, vitamin B12		Occasional
• Hypogeusesthesia, hyposmia	Zinc		Occasional
• Swollen, retracted, bleeding gums (if teeth are present)	Vitamin C		Occasional
Bones, Joints			
• Beading of ribs, epiphyseal swelling, bowlegs	Vitamin D		Rare
• Tenderness (subperiosteal hemorrhage in child)	Vitamin C		Rare
Neurologic			
• Headache		Vitamin A	Rare
• Drowsiness, lethargy, vomiting		Vitamins A, D	Rare
• Dementia	Niacin, vitamin B12		Rare
• Confabulation, disorientation	Thiamine (Korsakoff's psychosis)		Occasional
• Ophthalmoplegia	Thiamine, phosphorus		Occasional
• Peripheral neuropathy	Thiamine, pyridoxine, vitamin B12	Pyridoxine	Occasional
• Tetany	Calcium, magnesium		Occasional
Other			
• Parotid enlargement	Protein (also consider bulimia)		Occasional
• Heart failure	Thiamine (wet beriberi), phosphorus		Occasional
• Sudden heart failure, death	Vitamin C		Rare
• Hepatomegaly	Protein	Vitamin A	Rare
• Edema	Protein, thiamine		Common
• Poor healing wounds, decubitus ulcers	Protein, vitamin C, zinc		Common

IV. ENERGY AND PROTEIN REQUIREMENTS FOR ADULT PATIENTS

METABOLIC RESPONSE TO STRESS

The metabolic response to stress or injury (e.g., sepsis, organ failure, severe thermal injury, severe trauma, major surgery) is typically seen in critically ill patients. Stress is associated with hypermetabolism and hypercatabolism, resulting in altered energy expenditure and breakdown of body energy stores (muscle proteins, glycogen, and fat). In the absence of adequate nutrition support, patients under stress may develop protein-energy malnutrition. Malnourished patients have decreased immune systems, and malnutrition is associated with increased patient morbidity, mortality, and prolonged hospital stay.

During stress, there is increased sympathetic nervous system stimulation, leading to increased production of counter-regulatory hormones (e.g., catecholamines, cortisol, glucagon, growth hormone) and release of cytokines (e.g., tumor necrosis factor-α, interleukins 1 and 6) and other immune mediators such as thromboxanes (TXA2) and prostaglandins (PGFα, PGE2). The end-results are accelerated proteolysis, glycogenolysis, lipolysis, gluconeogenesis, insulin resistance, and hyperglycemia. Additionally, amino acid transport into skeletal muscles is impaired, which is coupled with proteolysis leading to negative nitrogen balance and weight loss. Stressed patients have reduced tolerance to carbohydrates that may result in hyperglycemia, and have reduced fat utilization that may lead to hypertriglyceridemia.

Despite increased calorie and protein requirements, nutrient metabolism is altered during acute illness. Nutrition support therapy should balance calorie and protein intake to the body's metabolic capacities in order to ensure efficient nutrients utilization. It is essential to accurately estimate or measure the patient's calorie and protein requirements, avoid overfeeding (and potentially beneficial is short-term permissive underfeeding), and closely monitor the patient's response to nutrition support therapy. Adjustments to nutrition support therapy should mainly be guided by the patient's tolerance, rather than solely relying on the calorie and protein requirement estimates or measures.

ENERGY REQUIREMENTS

Estimating Energy Requirements

Basal energy expenditure (BEE) or basal metabolic rate (BMR) describes the metabolic activity required to maintain life (i.e., respiration, heart rate, body temperature, and other essential functions). Nearly 200 equations are available to predict energy expenditure, but no single equation accurately predicts energy expenditure in most hospitalized patients. There is also debate over the best energy predictive equation and what body weight should be used in obese individuals (body mass index, BMI $\geq$ 30 kg/m^2) to determine energy requirements.

The 2002 American Society for Parenteral and Enteral Nutrition (A.S.P.E.N.) guidelines for the use of parenteral and enteral nutrition state that the estimated calorie requirements for adult patients generally range from 20 to 35 kcal/kg/day.

The most widely used energy predictive equations are the Harris-Benedict equations that account for sex, weight, height, and age for estimating the BEE, although they are skewed to young, non-obese individuals:

Men   BEE = 66 + (13.7 x W) + (5 x H) - (6.8 x A)

Women   BEE = 655 + (9.6 x W) + (1.7 x H) - (4.7 x A)

W = weight (kg); H = height (cm); A = age (years)

Conversions: 1 kg = 2.2 lb; 1 ft = 12 in; 1 in = 2.54 cm

The resting energy expenditure (REE) or resting metabolic rate (RMR) is the amount of calories required by the body during 24 hours in a non-active state. REE is approximately 10% higher than the BEE because it adjusts for the thermic effect of food and the awake state. Total energy expenditure (TEE) to maintain current body weight is estimated by multiplying the BEE by the appropriate "activity" factor based on activity level and/or anabolic status, as follows:

Bed rest/sedentary   1.2 x BEE
Ambulatory   1.3 x BEE
Anabolic   1.5 x BEE

Alternatively, the patient's calorie goal can be calculated by multiplying the BEE (calculated from the Harris-Benedict equations) by a "stress" or "injury" factor ranging from 1.2 to 1.5, depending on the severity of injury or the patient's stress level. For instance, a stress factor of 1.2 can be applied to the case of a non-malnourished adult patient following minor surgery. A higher stress factor of 1.4 to 1.5 may be applied to the case of an adult patient with ongoing sepsis, severe thermal injury, or with a history of severe malnutrition.

Energy requirements are increased 12% with each degree of fever over 37^0 Celsius.

Conversions: 9 x T (degree Celsius) = 5 x T (degree Fahrenheit) – 160

T = body temperature

The RMR in critically ill, non-obese, mechanically ventilated, adult patients can be calculated using the Penn State equations:

$$RMR = (0.85 \times BEE) + (33 \times V_E) + (175 \times T_{max}) - 6433$$

$$RMR = (0.96 \times BMR) + (31 \times V_E) + (167 \times T_{max}) - 6212$$

BEE calculated using Harris-Benedict equations
BMR calculated using Mifflin-St. Jeor equation
V_E = minute ventilation (L/min); T_{max} = maximum body temperature (degrees Celsius)

The debate surrounding the use of actual body weight or adjusted body weight to estimate the RMR in obese individuals is partly related to estimating the fat mass and fat-free mass of body weight; their relation to energy expenditure, age, and gender; and the fat mass that is metabolically active. Recommendations for adjustments ranged between 25% and 50% (i.e., multiplying by factors between 0.25 and 0.5), implying that 25% to 50% of the fat mass is metabolically active in an obese person. Current recommendations are to use an adjusted body weight of 50% of the difference between the ideal body weight (IBW) and actual body weight in the Harris-Benedict equations in patients with BMI between 30 and 50 kg/m^2, with a "stress" factor of 1.3 for estimating TEE. The adjusted body weight is calculated as follows:

Adjusted body weight = IBW + (actual body weight – IBW) x 0.5

IBW = ideal body weight

The IBW is a theoretical weight estimate based on height and frame size. Table 1 shows the methods of estimating the IBW.

Table 1. Estimated Weight Allowance for Height to Calculate the Ideal Body Weight

Build	Women	Men
Medium	Allow 100 lb (45.5 kg) for first 5 ft (152.4 cm) of height plus 5 lb (2.3 kg) for each additional inch (2.5 cm)	Allow 106 lb (48.2 kg) for first 5 ft (152.4 cm) of height plus 6 lb (2.7 kg) for each additional inch (2.5 cm)
Small	Subtract 10%	Subtract 10%
Large	Add 10%	Add 10%

Reprinted with modifications from: Committees of the American Diabetes Association, Inc. and the American Dietetic Association, 1977. A guide for professionals: the effective application of exchange lists for meal planning, p. 17.

The BMR for overweight and obese, non-critically ill, hospitalized adult patients can be predicted using the following Mifflin-St. Jeor equations:

Men $\qquad$ $BMR = (10 \times W) + (6.25 \times H) - (5 \times A) + 5$

Women $\qquad$ $BMR = (10 \times W) + (6.25 \times H) - (5 \times A) - 161$

W = weight (kg); H = height (cm); A = age (years)

Measuring Energy Expenditure

The variability in energy expenditure and lack of accurate energy predicting equations for critically ill patients make indirect calorimetry a valuable tool to assess the RMR that reflects the patient's clinical condition. Indirect calorimetry measures the volume of oxygen consumption (VO_2) and carbon dioxide production (VCO_2). In critically ill patients, calories are provided at 100% to 130% of the RMR. Indirect calorimetry provides a measure of the respiratory quotient (RQ), which is the ratio between VCO_2 and VO_2. The RQ should be used as an indicator of indirect calorimetry validity and not an indicator of substrate utilization. If the RQ exceeds 1, this could be an indication of overfeeding and lipogenesis. The corresponding RQ for oxidized substrates is 0.7 for fat, 0.8 for proteins, and 1 for carbohydrates.

Energy expenditure measurements using indirect calorimetry are routinely performed by the Metabolic Laboratory clinicians twice weekly in our hospital selected intensive care units (SICU, BICU, CCMU) for critically ill patients who meet specific criteria and conditions (e.g., mechanically ventilated patients; $FiO_2 \leq 0.6$; patient undisturbed for at least 30 minutes before measurements; wait of at least 4 hours after hemodialysis and at least 1 hour after ventilator changes; absence of air leak from chest and endotracheal tubes or ventilator circuit). For patients on other services, an order can be placed in CareLink (Computerized Prescriber Order Entry, CPOE) as "REE" for energy expenditure measurement. The Metabolic Laboratory Service can be reached 24/7 (pager 2349) or by paging the Metabolic Laboratory Service Clinical Specialist on weekdays (pager 3296).

PROTEIN REQUIREMENTS

There is no consensus on the body weight (actual, ideal, or adjusted) to use for protein requirements in adult patients. Some practices base protein requirements on IBW for normally nourished patients and actual body weight for malnourished patients. Expert opinion suggests that protein requirements be based on actual body weight for normal body-sized or malnourished patients and using IBW for obese patients (Table 2).

Table 2. Daily Protein Requirements Based on Clinical Condition for Adult Patients

Clinical conditions	Protein requirements (g/kg)[a]
Maintenance, Non-stressed	1–1.2
Repletion	1.3–2
Trauma, Thermal injury, Neurotrauma	1.5–2
Hepatic encephalopathy	0.8–1.2
Liver failure without encephalopathy	1.2–1.5
Peridialysis (Acute kidney injury, Chronic kidney disease)	0.8–1
Intermittent hemodialysis, Peritoneal dialysis	1.2–1.5
Continuous Renal Replacement Therapy (CRRT)	1.5–2.5[b]

[a]Use ideal body weight for obese patients. Protein requirements vary, and should be adjusted based
on underlying diseases, clinical conditions, nutritional status, and tolerance.
[b]Based on clinical studies, amino acid losses across the CRRT hemodiafilter can be estimated at about 0.2 g/kg/day. This amount varies with plasma amino acid concentrations and hemodiafiltration rate.

PERMISSIVE UNDERFEEDING

Permissive underfeeding refers to providing nutrition support to critically ill, metabolically stressed, adult patients with calories less than their daily requirements for a short time, to avoid exacerbation of the metabolic response to stress. It is reasonable to aim at providing permissive underfeeding at about 80% of daily energy requirements especially with parenteral nutrition, although lesser daily calories have been provided in clinical studies of permissive underfeeding. Lower calorie intake may be beneficial by avoiding carbohydrate loading that could result in hyperglycemia, increased carbon dioxide production, and hepatic steatosis. Providing additional calories, even with sufficient protein intake, does not attenuate hypercatabolism in metabolically stressed, critically ill patients. In fact, the metabolic rate of most critically ill patients is not always significantly increased, and excessive calories result in substantial body fat gain relative to nitrogen retention.

There is little evidence that meeting predictive or measured energy requirements is of clinical benefit or improves patient outcomes. Rather, providing nutrition support therapy below energy requirements may decrease patient ventilator dependence, length of hospital stay, and antibiotic use. However, compelling evidence to support permissive underfeeding is lacking, and there are concerns that underfeeding and energy deficit may increase infection rate and negatively affect patient outcome.

The optimal amounts of calories for critically ill patients are not well defined. However, caloric intake at less than 25% of energy requirements (based on the American College of Chest Physicians guidelines) was associated with significantly increased rate of bloodstream infections in medicine intensive care unit patients. Prospective randomized controlled studies are needed to prove the safety and efficacy of permissive underfeeding. Inappropriate underfeeding or overfeeding can have additional adverse consequences in critically ill patients.

HYPOCALORIC FEEDING

Hypocaloric feeding is defined as the provision of high-protein and low-calorie EN or PN to obese patients (BMI $\geq$ 30) to achieve net protein anabolism, avoid the complications of excessive calorie intake and exacerbation of metabolic stress, avoid body fat weight gain, and possibly promote fat weight loss. The obese patient is at high risk for insulin resistance, hyperglycemia, poor surgical wound healing, and postoperative infectious complications, and may have protein depletion with decreased muscle mass. In clinical studies, caloric intake with hypocaloric feeding of obese and morbidly obese patients has ranged from 11 to 14 kcal/kg/day of actual body weight, or about 22 to 25 kcal/kg/day of IBW, with protein intake at 2 to 2.5 g/kg of IBW (in the absence of renal or liver failure). Hypocaloric feeding should be adjusted based on the patient's clinical response with the primary goal of achieving net protein anabolism. The minimal amount of adequate calories is not well established and there are concerns of inducing ketoacidosis with starvation. Hypocaloric feeding has not been evaluated in patients with kidney injury, liver disease and hepatic encephalopathy, and the optimal duration, safety, and efficacy of hypocaloric feeding in critically ill obese patients remain unknown.

V. ENTERAL NUTRITION FOR ADULT AND ADOLESCENT PATIENTS

Enteral nutrition (EN) refers to the administration of nutrients for a therapeutic purpose through a tube into the gastrointestinal tract. Nasoenteric or enterostomy tube feedings are indicated when patients are unable to ingest sufficient nutrients by mouth. A functional gastrointestinal tract is necessary for successful EN. The length and absorptive capacity of the intestines dictate the volume, type, and choice of enteral feeding and EN formula(s).

EN is contraindicated in the presence of intestinal obstruction, paralytic ileus, active upper gastrointestinal hemorrhage, intractable diarrhea, unstable hypotension, and certain small bowel fistulae when feeding below the fistula is contraindicated.

EN has key advantages compared to parenteral nutrition (PN) that include:
- Maintaining gut integrity, preventing gut villi atrophy, stimulating gut villi development, preserving gut-associated lymphoid tissue (GALT), and restoring gastrointestinal function
- Lower rate of infectious complications
- Lower incidence of hyperglycemia
- Reduced risk of cholestasis, cholelithiasis, and biliary sludge
- Less expensive

Early EN in critically ill patients within 24 to 48 hours of admission to the intensive care unit decreases infectious complications, modulates oxidative stress and systemic immune responses, attenuates disease severity, and may shorten the length of intensive care unit stay. Early EN following gastrointestinal surgery may also decrease the risk of infections and reduce the length of hospital stay.

ENTERAL NUTRITION FORMULAS

EN formulas (except infant formulas) are considered "medical foods," and are not regulated by the Food and Drug Administration (FDA). Medical foods fall under the regulations that apply to good manufacturing practices (GMP), and regulations that ensure the sterility of low-acid, thermally processed foods. They are exempt from regulations on labeling and health claims such as those that apply to medications.

Key elements considered when selecting an EN formula include formula caloric density, protein content, fat content, osmolality, and nutrient complexity. Enteral modular supplements are also available to provide additional supplements to standard EN formulas. The addition of modular supplements alters the caloric distribution in the formula and results in a more concentrated formula with higher osmolality that may negatively impact feeding tolerance. Contact the registered dietitian on service for assistance with the choice of modular supplements and appropriateness for mixing and delivery of EN formulas.

Refer to Appendix B and the Patient Food and Nutrition Services internal website (http://www.med.umich.edu/i/pfans/), which provide descriptive listing of adult EN formulas available on Formulary.

Caloric Density

Adult EN formulas have a caloric density ranging from 1 to 2 kcal/mL. A 2 kcal/mL formula is indicated for patients who require fluid restriction.

Protein

EN formulas available on Formulary contain 4% to 22% of total calories as protein. Most commonly used sources of protein include soy protein isolates, casein, whey, lactoalbumin, and crystalline amino acids. Protein equivalency of these sources is nutritionally comparable, and various sources can be interchanged. Chemically defined EN formulas that contain enzymatically hydrolyzed proteins are available for patients with malabsorption syndromes. High nitrogen EN formulas are useful for patients with increased catabolic demands (e.g., trauma) or increased nitrogen losses (e.g., severe thermal injury).

Carbohydrate

Common sources of carbohydrates in EN formulas include maltodextrin, corn syrup, and cornstarch. All commercial EN formulas are lactose-free to avoid lactose intolerance especially in critically ill patients who may have reduced lactase production.

Fat

Fat in EN formulas available on Formulary constitute 4% to 40% of total calories. Primary fat sources are from vegetable oils including corn, safflower, sunflower, canola, and soy oil. These fat sources provide mostly long-chain triglycerides (LCT) and are generally equally tolerated. Some products contain a higher percentage of fat as medium-chain triglycerides (MCT). MCT are beneficial in patients with malabsorption syndromes because they do not require pancreatic lipase or bile for intestinal absorption. However, MCT (C6 to C12) lack the essential fatty acids (i.e., linoleic acid, α-linolenic acid) that are part of the long-chain fatty acids (C18).

Fibers

Predominantly insoluble fibers (e.g., soy polysaccharide) are added to certain EN formulas to increase stool volume, prevent constipation, and reduce intestinal transit time. Insoluble fibers are generally poorly fermentable and reach the large intestine mostly intact.

Some EN formulas may contain soluble fibers (e.g., guar gum, pectin) that may improve glucose tolerance and may have trophic effects on the ileal and colonic mucosa. Soluble fibers are generally highly fermentable. They partially dissolve in the upper gastrointestinal tract to form a gel-like substance that causes delay in gastric emptying. Soluble fibers also absorb water in the intestines to form a viscous liquid that induces peristalsis and reduces intestinal transit time.

Water

EN formulas that provide 1 kcal/mL are about 85% water. EN formulas that provide 2 kcal/mL are about 70% water, and are indicated for patients who require fluid restriction.

Osmolality

Osmolality is a measure of the oncotic pressure exerted by a solution and is expressed as mOsm/kg of water. Soluble minerals and carbohydrates primarily determine the osmolality of the EN formula. Isotonic EN formulas (osmolality of 350 mOsm/kg) should be selected for the transition interval whenever possible.

Nutrient Complexity

Some EN formulas provide nutrients in readily absorbable elemental forms (e.g., monosaccharides, disaccharides, amino acids, dipeptides, tripeptides, medium-chain triglycerides, and long-chain triglycerides). These formulas have minimal residue, low viscosity, but have high osmolality. Because of their elemental composition, these formulas do not elicit the same degree of intestinal secretory response compared to complex EN formulas. The use of elemental EN formulas during the transition from PN to EN results in decreased levels of digestive enzymes and secretions that are known to stimulate mucosal growth and regeneration, which may result in decreased EN tolerance. Clinical studies have not yet demonstrated the superiority of elemental EN formulas compared to intact protein formulas. Patients with enterocutaneous fistulae may benefit from elemental EN formulas that may reduce enteric secretions.

IMMUNONUTRITION AND IMMUNE–MODULATING NUTRIENTS

Growing evidence suggests that specific nutrients or combinations of these nutrients may enhance immune function in certain patient populations. The so-called "immune-modulating nutrients" include L-glutamine, L-arginine, nucleic acids, omega-3 fatty acids (eicosapentanoic acid, EPA and docosahexaenoic acid, DHA), and antioxidants. L–glutamine is considered a conditionally essential or indispensable amino acid under conditions of metabolic stress. It is preferentially used as a fuel source in cells that replicate rapidly such as gastrointestinal mucosal cells and immune cells (e.g. macrophages and lymphocytes). L–arginine is also considered a conditionally essential or indispensable amino acid and may improve immune response and wound healing. Nucleotides are required for many metabolic processes and may also be important to rapidly growing and replicating cells. Omega-3 fatty acids are precursors of the three-series eicosanoids and five-series leukotrienes. These eicosanoids and leukotrienes promote decreased inflammation and immune suppression better than the two-series eicosanoids and four-series leukotrienes (products of omega-6 fatty acid metabolism via cyclooxygenase). The administration of omega-3 fatty acids alters the composition of cell membranes and decreases the ratio of omega-6 to omega-3 fatty acids. This may increase the synthesis of eicosanoids and leukotrienes that have beneficial effect on inflammation and the immune system.

Clinical studies that evaluated the immune modulating EN products, containing one or a combination of immune modulating nutrients, have shown that specific patient populations may have fewer infectious complications, shorter days on mechanical ventilation, and shorter length of stay in the intensive care unit. Limitations to the studies include a small number of patients, reported conflicting results, and the effect on mortality has not been consistently demonstrated. Further, the cost of these immune modulating EN products can be significantly higher than standard EN products. Routine clinical use of immune modulating formulas cannot be recommended until further data clearly demonstrate their benefit and cost-efficacy.

The American Society for Parenteral and Enteral Nutrition (A.S.P.E.N.) and Society for Critical Care Medicine (SCCM) issued in the year 2009 the Critical Care Guidelines for nutrition support practice in critically ill patients. The guidelines state that immune modulating EN formulations should be used only for appropriate patient population including patients following major elective surgery, trauma, thermal injury, head and neck cancer, and critically ill patients on mechanical ventilation. Critically ill patients with adult respiratory distress syndrome (ARDS) and severe acute lung injury should receive EN formulas providing anti-inflammatory lipids (e.g., omega-3 fish oils, borage oil) and antioxidants. Glutamine addition to the EN regimen was also suggested to be considered in thermal injury, severe trauma, and mixed intensive care unit patients. At least 50% to 65% of daily energy requirements were believed to be necessary to be provided from the immune modulating formulas in order to achieve therapeutic benefits. The guidelines caution about the use of immune modulating formulas in patients with severe sepsis.

The immune modulating EN formulas available on Formulary are Crucial® and Oxepa®. Crucial® is a peptide-based elemental formula with a caloric density of 1.5 kcal/mL and provides proteins 94 g/L. It contains immune-modulating nutrients of combined DHA and EPA 4.3 g/L and arginine 15 g/L. It also contains high amounts of beta-carotene, vitamin A, vitamin C, and zinc. Crucial® is not restricted for use in critically ill patients, but its use is limited to patients who are likely to benefit most from its use. These include patients with blunt and penetrating torso trauma and those undergoing elective gastrointestinal surgery (benefit most likely in malnourished patients).

Oxepa® contains EPA 4.6 g/L and gamma-linolenic acid 4 g/L, with increased amounts of antioxidants (vitamins E and C, beta-carotene) and taurine. Gamma-linolenic acid is believed to produce less inflammatory eicosanoids with increased production of prostaglandin E_1, a pulmonary vasodilator that improves circulation, gas exchange, and oxygenation. Oxepa® is restricted for use in pediatric and adult intensive care units for patients who meet specific criteria of acute respiratory distress syndrome, or acute lung injury. More information about EN and the coordination of requests and use of specialized EN formulas can be obtained by contacting the registered dietitian on service, or by checking the Patient Food and Nutrition Services internal website http://www.med.umich.edu/i/pfans/.

MONITORING ENTERAL NUTRITION

Most complications related to the administration of EN can be easily treated and prevented through proper monitoring and intervention. During enteral feeding administration, the patient should be monitored for nausea, diarrhea, abdominal cramping, and bloating (Chapters VII and XI).

ORAL MEDICATION ADMINISTRATION WITH ENTERAL NUTRITION

Whenever possible, medications should be administered orally to prevent feeding tube occlusion. Otherwise, medications should be obtained in oral liquid forms whenever possible to facilitate medication administration through the feeding tube. Elixirs and oral suspensions should be diluted with water before administration via the feeding tube. Each medication should be administered separately. The feeding tube should be flushed with 5 to 10 mL of warm water after each medication is administered and prior to restarting feeding.

Oral medications that should not be crushed include sublingual, buccal, enteric-coated, and extended-release products. In addition, some preparations should not be crushed because they can cause irritation to the oral mucosa, are extremely bitter, or could stain teeth. A list of oral dosage forms that should not be crushed (Appendix F) is generated and updated by the Institute for Safe Medication Practice (ISMP) and can be accessed electronically at http://www.ismp.org/Tools/DoNotCrush.pdf.

FOOD-DRUG INTERACTIONS

Food-drug interactions usually occur with oral diets, but some significant drug-nutrient interactions may also occur with tube feeding. Key food-drug interactions are shown in Appendix G. Food-drug interactions policy (07-01-035), list of key food-drug interactions and patient education material are found at the internal web link
http://www.med.umich.edu/i/policies/umh/07-01-035.html.

VI. PARENTERAL NUTRITION FOR ADOLESCENT AND ADULT PATIENTS

Establishing the proper indication for PN and obtaining appropriate venous access are the first steps before selecting a PN formulation. PN should be limited to patients with intestinal failure, bowel obstruction, high output enterocutaneous fistula(e), and prolonged ileus. There are no clinical benefits to supplementing EN with PN, unless in the long-term home PN patient. If PN is indicated, a systematic approach is followed to formulate PN, to ensure the efficacy and safety of PN therapy. PN is designed by considering the patient's clinical condition(s), nutritional status, fluid volume status, laboratory data, and medication therapy. A balanced PN formulation provides daily calories at 10% to 20% from amino acids, 20% to 30% from lipids, and 50% to 60% from dextrose, in addition to adequate vitamins, trace elements, electrolytes, and fluids.

MACRONUTRIENTS

Macronutrients are the energy-yielding substrates in PN and include amino acids, dextrose, and intravenous lipid emulsions.

Amino Acids

Amino acids are a source of nitrogen and are used for protein synthesis. Amino acids are provided in PN to restore or preserve lean body mass and visceral proteins, promote wound healing, and to improve or maintain nitrogen balance. Amino acids are a source of energy with a caloric value of 4 kcal/g. Adequate calories from dextrose and intravenous lipid emulsions must be provided to optimize nitrogen retention.

The two parenteral amino acid bulk solutions on Formulary for use in the PN of adolescent and adult patients are FreAmine III[®] 10% and Aminosyn II[®] 15%. FreAmine III[®] 10% is the parenteral amino acid bulk solution of choice for adult and adolescent patients. A key difference between these two parenteral amino acid formulations is their inherent electrolyte content, essentially the inherent phosphate 10 mmol/L in FreAmine III[®] 10%. Aminosyn II[®] 15% contains no phosphate and is restricted for use in patients with persistent hyperphosphatemia despite restriction of oral or parenteral phosphate intake. CareLink (Computerized Prescriber Order Entry, CPOE) automatically calculates the total electrolyte content based on the amounts and types of amino acid solutions used in PN formulations. The parenteral crystalline amino acid bulk solutions available on Formulary are shown in Appendix H.

To determine protein requirements for adult patients, refer to Chapter IV. In CareLink, amino acids in the final adult PN admixture are reported as "g/kg", "per day" amounts, percent of final PN volume, and percent of total daily calories in PN. Compounding limits of amino acids in PN are shown in Table 1.

Dextrose

Hydrous dextrose (d-glucose) is the major source of immediate energy that yields 3.4 kcal/g, and a source of carbon skeletons essential for tissue growth and cellular metabolism. Generally, a dextrose infusion rate of 2 mg/kg/min per 24 hours is optimal to suppress gluconeogenesis, and provides adequate protein-sparing effect in adult patients. Glucose utilization decreases with advancing age, diabetes, liver disease, sepsis, stress, and medication therapy (e.g., corticosteroids, tacrolimus). Maximal continuous dextrose infusion rate in stressed adult patients should not exceed 4 mg/kg/min to minimize the risk of hyperglycemia and reduce insulin requirements. Calculation of dextrose infusion rate (DIR) is as follows:

$$DIR\ (mg/kg/min) = \frac{Total\ dextrose\ (mg)}{Body\ weight\ (kg)^a \times (1{,}440\ min)^b}$$

[a]Use adjusted body weight in obese patients
[b]24 hours = 1,440 minutes

In CareLink, dextrose in the final adult PN admixture is reported as "per day" amounts, percent of final PN volume, percent of total daily calories in PN, and as dextrose infusion rate (mg/kg/min) for a 24 hour-infusion. Compounding limits of dextrose in PN are shown in Table 1.

Table 1. Maximum Amino Acid and Dextrose Concentrations in Adult Parenteral Nutrition Admixtures

Parenteral nutrition admixture	Central			Peripheral
Amino acid concentration (per 1000 mL)	42.5 g	50 g	60 g	25 g
Dextrose concentration (per 1000 mL)	350 g	300 g	250 g	100 g

Intravenous Lipid Emulsions

Intravenous lipid emulsion particles are similar in size to chylomicrons (0.5 micron), but lack apoproteins (polypeptides that activate enzyme systems) on their external coating. Lipid particles acquire apoproteins on their coating in the bloodstream, which facilitates their metabolism by the lipoprotein lipase enzyme. Lipid particles are then hydrolyzed by the lipoprotein lipase to free fatty acids, which are then stored as triglycerides in adipose tissue, or oxidized to adenosine triphosphate (ATP). The remaining fatty acids circulate in the bloodstream bound to albumin. Fatty acid remnants are metabolized in the liver by the liver lipase enzyme to very-low-density lipoproteins (VLDL) and ATP. High concentrations of lipids in the bloodstream may overwhelm the lipoprotein lipase activity that can result in hypertriglyceridemia. The plasma half-life of intravenous lipid emulsions is about 30 minutes. Under normal conditions, plasma lipid clearance occurs within 80 minutes, with 80% cleared in one hour.

Intravenous lipid emulsions are a source of calories and essential fatty acids (linoleic acid, α-linolenic acid). Intravenous lipid emulsions in the United States are composed of long-chain fatty acids. They are commercially available as 10%, 20%, and 30% weight by volume oil-in-water emulsions that yield 1.1, 2, and 3 kcal/mL, respectively.

The phospholipid-to-triglyceride ratios in the Liposyn® products is 0.12 for the 10% intravenous lipid emulsion, and 0.06 for the 20% and 30% emulsions. The lower phospholipid amount in the 20% and 30% compared to the 10% emulsion favors a better lipid clearance, and makes the 20% and 30% intravenous lipid emulsions favored over the 10% emulsion in patients with reduced lipid clearance (e.g., critically ill patients). Accumulation of cholesterol, triglycerides, and phospholipids in the form of an abnormal lipoprotein X occurs with the 10% emulsion infusion. Lipoprotein X particles have a long half-life, are slowly cleared from the bloodstream, and may compete with triglycerides for clearance. Lipoprotein X may then contribute to the elevation of serum triglyceride concentrations, especially in patients with predisposing factors to hypertriglyceridemia.

The 20% intravenous lipid emulsion is the only available on Formulary (Table 2). The PN admixture is compounded as 2-in-1 admixture with intravenous lipid emulsions administered at the "Y" connector tubing. The 30% lipid emulsion is approved only for use in preparing total nutrient admixtures (TNA) or 3-in-1 PN admixtures and is not on Formulary.

Intravenous lipid emulsions usually provide 20% to 30% of total daily calories in PN. The typical intravenous lipid emulsion dose in adults should not exceed 1 g/kg/day. To prevent essential fatty acid deficiency, adult patients should be provided with a minimum of about 2% to 4% of total daily calories from linoleic acid, which is equivalent to about 500 mL weekly or 250 mL biweekly infusion of 20% intravenous lipid emulsion. Plasma essential fatty acid profile should be regularly monitored (e.g., every 2 to 3 months) whenever intravenous lipid emulsion infusion or oral fat intake is restricted.

Intravenous lipid emulsions are isotonic solutions that can be infused safely through a peripheral vein without the risk of phlebitis. Co-infusing lipid emulsions with PN also reduces the overall PN admixture osmolarity, thereby reducing phlebitis risk.

Table 2. Intravenous Lipid Emulsion

Liposyn III® 20%	
Fat sources	Soybean oil
Total fat (%)	20
Fatty acids (%)[a]	
Linoleic acid[a,b]	54.5
Oleic acid	22.4
Palmitic acid	10.5
Linolenic acid[b]	8.3
Stearic acid	4.2
Egg phosphatides[c] (%)	1.2
Glycerin[d] (%)	2.5
Caloric density[e]	2 kcal/mL
Osmolarity	292 mOsm/L
pH	8.3 (6–9)
Phospholipids-to-triglycerides ratio	0.06

[a]Of the total fat calories, 1.1 kcal/mL is supplied by linoleic acid.
[b]Essential fatty acids.
[c]Egg yolk phospholipids added as emulsifiers. Intravenous lipid emulsions provide approximately 7.5 millimoles of phosphates per each 500 mL.
[d]Glycerin added to adjust tonicity.
[e]Includes calories from glycerol, egg phosphatides, and fat.

Allergic reactions that may occur with intravenous lipid emulsion infusion can be related to rapid lipid infusion rate or cross-sensitivity in patients with allergy to eggs or legumes (e.g., broad beans, soy beans, lentils). The infusion rate of intravenous lipid emulsions should not exceed 0.12 g/kg per hour. Infusion-related adverse effects associated may include fever, chills, headache, nausea, dyspnea, chest tightness, and palpitations. Intravenous lipid emulsions are safe to use in patients with chylothorax and chylous ascites, and do not increase chyle volume because they are metabolized by the lipoprotein lipase enzyme into fatty acids in the bloodstream.

Intravenous lipid emulsions and the immune system

Soybean oil-based intravenous lipid emulsions have been the standard intravenous lipid emulsions used in PN. Concerns have been raised about the possibility that these emulsions interfere with immune function and possibly increase infectious complications. Soybean oil-based intravenous lipid emulsions provide high amounts of omega-6 fatty acids, essentially linoleic acid (C18:2ω-6), and long-chain polyunsaturated fatty acids that are considered proinflammatory with possible immunomodulating effects, and may pose the risk for infectious complications. Further, exposure to large amounts of long-chain polyunsaturated fatty acids may increase cell membrane peroxidation that may further cause oxidative stress in critically ill patients. The American Society for Parenteral and Enteral Nutrition (A.S.P.E.N.) and Society for Critical Care Medicine (SCCM) 2009 Critical Care Guidelines state that omega-6 fatty acids-based intravenous lipid emulsions should not be given to critically ill patients receiving PN during their first week in the intensive care unit (grade D recommendation, i.e., supported by at least two level III investigations).

Intravenous lipid emulsions containing fish oil or olive oil have been suggested to replace soybean-based lipid emulsions. Fish oil provides omega-3 fatty acids that are less proinflammatory than the omega-6 fatty acids. Olive oil-based intravenous lipid emulsions are rich in the long-chain monounsaturated oleic acid (C18:1ω-9) that would avoid the high intake of linoleic acid.

Data from large prospective randomized controlled studies are needed to further evaluate the role of omega-3 fatty acids-based lipid emulsions. Because hyperglycemia is detrimental to the immune system and predisposes patients to increased infectious complications, glycemic control (e.g., serum glucose concentrations between 110 to 150 mg/dl) with continuous insulin infusion is essential. EN is associated with fewer infectious complications compared to PN and should be used in preference to PN.

FLUIDS

Fluids in PN are ordered as "per day" amounts. PN should not be used to replace acute fluid losses. It is clinically more appropriate and cost-effective to correct fluid losses with appropriate intravenous fluids (Appendix I). Guidelines for estimating maintenance fluid requirements based on body weight are shown in Table 3.

Table 3. Estimation of Maintenance Fluid Requirements[a]

Body Weight	Fluid
$\leq$ 10 kg	100 mL/kg/day
10–20 kg	1000 mL + 50 mL for each kg over 10 kg
> 20 kg	1500 mL + 20 mL for each kg over 20 kg

[a]For every degree increase in body temperature over 38^0 C (100.4^0 F), about 10% more fluid above maintenance requirements should be administered.

A patient's fluid intake and losses (e.g., gastrointestinal, urinary) should be continuously recorded. Reducing PN volume may be indicated in oliguric (urine losses < 400 mL/day) and anuric (urine losses < 50 mL/day) patients, and in those with congestive heart failure. PN-dependent patients with chronic fluid losses from the upper (e.g., gastric losses with suctioning, vomiting) or lower (e.g., diarrhea, high-output ileostomy, enterocutaneous fistulae) gastrointestinal tract can have a portion or all of their maintenance and replacement fluid requirements included in PN admixtures.

ELECTROLYTES

Electrolytes are essential for the proper functioning of biochemical reactions and homeostatic functions. They are involved in maintaining cell membrane functions, enzymatic and hormonal activities, nerve conductivity, cardiovascular function, muscle contractility, bone structure, and fluid and acid-base homeostasis.

Electrolytes are supplemented in PN admixtures as amounts "per day" in the form of salts including sodium chloride or acetate, potassium chloride or acetate, phosphorus as sodium or potassium phosphate, calcium gluconate, and magnesium sulfate. For safety, stability, and compounding reasons, specific limits are set for the maximum concentrations and amounts of electrolytes that can be added in PN. Acute electrolyte deficiencies should be corrected with electrolyte supplementation outside the PN in order to achieve a timely and clinically effective correction of serum electrolyte concentrations.

There are no definitive recommendations for the exact dosing of electrolytes, and recommendations are largely based on evidence derived from studies, case reports, expert opinion, and clinical experience. Electrolyte supplementation is mainly guided by the patient's serum electrolyte concentrations, underlying clinical conditions, organ function (e.g., renal function, gastrointestinal losses), medication therapy (e.g., medications that cause electrolyte losses, retention, or shifts across cell membranes), acid-base status (e.g., acidemia and alkalemia have opposite effects on potassium shifts between compartments, and on calcium binding to albumin), and nutritional status (e.g., increased requirements during anabolism for potassium, phosphate, and magnesium). Sound clinical assessment, knowledge of the underlying pathophysiology of electrolyte imbalances, and an understanding of the consequences of electrolyte deficiencies and toxicities are essential for guiding electrolyte supplementation.

The typical ranges for maintenance electrolyte supplementation in PN admixtures are shown in Table 4. A summary of the key physiologic functions of electrolytes is shown in Table 5.

Table 4. Daily Electrolytes Maintenance Requirements and Concentration Limits in Parenteral Nutrition for Adult Patients

Electrolyte	Daily maintenance requirements	Concentration limit (per 1000 mL)
Sodium[a,b]	1–2 mEq/kg	154 mEq
Potassium	1–2 mEq/kg	20 mEq
Magnesium	8–24 mEq	20 mEq
Calcium	10–15 mEq	Variable[c]
Phosphorus[b]	20–40 mmol	Variable[c]
Chloride[b,d]	Variable[c]	Wide range[e]
Acetate[a,b,d]	Variable[c]	Wide range[e]

[a]Aminosyn II 15%® contains sodium 58.1 mEq/L and acetate 107.6 mEq/L of bulk amino acid solution.
[b]FreAmine III 10%® contains sodium 10 mEq/L, acetate 89 mEq/L, chloride < 3 mEq/L, and phosphate 10 mmol/L of bulk amino acid solution.
[c]Dependent on calcium and phosphate in-solution compatibility.
[d]Amounts vary with sodium and potassium added.
[e]Adjust as needed to maintain acid-base balance.

Table 5. Physiologic Functions of Electrolytes

Electrolyte	Physiologic functions
Sodium	Maintenance of extracellular fluid volume and tonicity; regulation of osmolarity and cell membrane potential
Potassium	Protein and glycogen synthesis; determination of resting membrane potential
Magnesium	Cofactor for many enzyme systems for transfer reactions involving ATP, muscle contractility, and nerve conduction
Calcium	Bone metabolism; blood coagulation; platelet adhesion; neuromuscular activity; endocrine and exocrine secretory functions; electrophysiology of heart and smooth muscles
Phosphorus	Source of ATP; essential for cell membranes, phosphoproteins, and nucleic acids; regulates carbohydrate, protein, and fat metabolism; regulates ammoniagenesis and glycolysis; required for 2,3 DPG formation in RBCs

ATP = adenosine triphosphate; DPG = diphosphoglycerate; RBCs = red blood cells.

Sodium

Sodium is the major extracellular cation, and serum sodium concentrations largely dictate plasma osmolality. Sodium can be added to PN as sodium chloride, acetate, or phosphate. One millimole of sodium phosphate yields 1.33 mEq of elemental sodium. Sodium chloride is the sodium salt added to

PN by default. For most patients with normal serum sodium concentration, it is reasonable to initiate PN with a sodium content at a 0.45% normal saline equivalent (i.e., about 77 mEq/L). Sodium in the PN admixture can be increased or decreased afterwards based on serum sodium concentrations and fluid status. In patients with bicarbonate deficit (e.g., diarrhea, high ileostomy fluid losses, acute kidney injury), a portion of sodium in PN can be provided as sodium acetate to help correct the bicarbonate deficit and restore the acid-base balance.

Potassium

Potassium is the major intracellular cation. Potassium chloride can be added to PN as potassium chloride, acetate, or phosphate. One millimole of potassium phosphate yields 1.47 mEq of elemental potassium. Because potassium is mainly eliminated via the kidneys, extreme caution should be used with potassium supplementation in patients with decreased kidney function. Potassium requirements are increased in patients treated with loop or thiazide diuretics, amphotericin B, micafungin, or voriconazole, and in those with high gastric and intestinal fluid losses. Potassium infusion rates in adult PN admixtures should not exceed 10 mEq/hr.

Magnesium

Magnesium is the second major intracellular cation. Magnesium in PN is added as magnesium sulfate. One gram of magnesium sulfate yields 8.1 mEq of elemental magnesium. Decreased kidney function causes magnesium accumulation. Common causes of hypomagnesemia include diarrhea, high ileostomy fluid losses, and medication therapy such as loop and thiazide diuretics, amphotericin B, voriconazole, tacrolimus, or cisplatin. Adequate correction of hypomagnesemia is essential for the correction of hypokalemia.

Calcium

Calcium is added to PN as calcium gluconate. One gram of calcium gluconate yields 4.56 mEq of elemental calcium. Calcium amounts that can be safely added in PN are dictated by the relative phosphate amounts in solution.

Phosphates

Phosphates can be added in PN as sodium or potassium phosphate. Because phosphorus availability is essential for generation of ATP (i.e., energy), a well-nourished patient with normal kidney function requires about 10 to 15 millimoles of phosphate per 1000 kcal to maintain normal serum phosphorus concentrations. At least about twice this amount of phosphorus is needed in malnourished patients with refeeding syndrome. Phosphorus is mainly excreted by the kidneys, and patients with decreased kidney function are at risk for hyperphosphatemia.

Chloride

Chloride is added to PN admixtures in the forms of sodium and potassium salts. Chloride is mainly eliminated via the kidneys. Serum chloride concentrations generally follow serum sodium concentrations as sodium and chloride are cation and anion pair. The chloride-to-acetate ratio is adjusted in the PN formulation based on the patient's acid-base status. Severe hyperchloremia (serum chloride concentration exceeding 130 mEq/L) may cause hyperchloremic metabolic acidosis.

Bicarbonate Precursors

Acetate is a bicarbonate precursor and is converted in vivo to bicarbonate at an equimolar basis. This conversion apparently occurs outside the liver, and is rapid but not immediate. High acetate infusion may cause metabolic alkalosis and possibly respiratory acidosis.

Gluconate (as calcium gluconate in PN admixtures) is a precursor of bicarbonate, but its effect on increasing serum bicarbonate concentrations is considered very minimal compared to the higher acetate amounts commonly added in PN admixtures.

Intravenous bicarbonate should never be added or co-infused with the PN admixture. Mixing bicarbonate with PN fluids may result in the release of carbon dioxide and the formation of insoluble calcium or magnesium carbonate salts.

Calcium-Phosphate Solubility

Patient reports of respiratory distress and fatalities were linked to the infusion of TNA with calcium-phosphate precipitates. The Food and Drug Administration (FDA) issued a safety alert in 1994 related to two patient deaths associated with calcium-phosphate precipitation in PN. Autopsy from these patients showed diffuse microvascular pulmonary emboli containing calcium-phosphate precipitates. Precipitates were masked by the opaque color of the TNA and where in-line filters were not used for PN infusion. To avoid calcium-phosphate in-solution precipitation, maximum amounts of calcium and phosphate allowed in PN admixtures at the University of Michigan Hospitals and Health Centers is calculated as follows:

Calcium (mEq/L) + Phosphate (mmol/L) $\leq$ 30/L of PN admixtures

Factors that affect calcium-phosphate precipitation include:

- Calcium and phosphate concentrations: solubility limits should guide the maximum limits for calcium and phosphate that should be added in PN admixtures
- Amino acid concentrations: the higher the concentrations of amino acids are, the lower the solution pH is, and more phosphate will likely bind to amino acids leaving less available phosphates to bind and precipitate with free calcium. Also, phosphate binding to amino acids leaves fewer free phosphates in solution to bind with calcium
- Solution pH: mainly determined by the final amino acid concentration. The lower the solution pH is, the lesser the risk for calcium-phosphate precipitation. Monobasic phosphates predominate at low pH; whereas, dibasic phosphates predominate at high pH, which makes less free dibasic phosphates available at low pH to bind the divalent calcium compared to the high pH environment
- Calcium salts: calcium gluconate is the preferred calcium salt in PN admixtures because it has a lower dissociation constant compared to calcium chloride, leaving less free calcium available in solution to bind phosphates
- Order of calcium and phosphate mixing: phosphorus is added first, followed by other PN components, then calcium is added last with frequent agitation of the PN admixture
- Temperature: when temperature increases, more calcium and phosphate dissociate in solution, and calcium-phosphate precipitation risk increases
- Storage time: more calcium and phosphate dissociate in solution over time, increasing the risk for calcium-phosphate binding and precipitation

When a 3-in-1 PN admixture is used, the PN calcium-phosphate compatibility should be calculated based on the PN volume that excludes intravenous lipid emulsions.

VITAMINS

Vitamins are essential micronutrients for substrate metabolism, body immunity, and tissue repair. Fat-soluble vitamins are primarily stored in fatty tissues and are not readily excreted. Consequently, deficiencies of vitamins A, D, E, and K develop slowly. With the exception of vitamin B12, water-soluble vitamins are not stored in significant amounts in the body, and their body stores may become rapidly depleted. Appendix A provides information on vitamin deficiencies, toxicities, monitoring, and supplementation. Table 6 provides the content of the parenteral adult multivitamin formulation on Formulary. This intravenous multivitamin product (Infuvite® Adult) provides 150 mcg of vitamin K in accordance with the FDA recommendations. Standard compounding of PN formulations include the use of intravenous multivitamins with vitamin K. A non-formulary parenteral adult multivitamin formulation without vitamin K can be made available for use in patients who develop resistance to warfarin despite warfarin dosage adjustments. Table 7 describes the known metabolic functions of vitamins.

Table 6. Composition and Dosing of Adult Intravenous Multivitamin

Vitamin	Infuvite® Adult (10 mL)
Fat-soluble vitamins	
Vitamin A (as palmitate)	3300 IU
Vitamin D3 (cholecalciferol)	200 IU (5 mcg)
Vitamin E (dl-alpha tocopheryl acetate)	10 IU (10 mg)
Vitamin K1 (phytonadione)	150 mcg
Water-soluble vitamins	
Thiamine (B1)	6 mg
Riboflavin (B2)	3.6 mg
Niacinamide (B3)	40 mg
Dexpanthenol (B5)	15 mg
Pyridoxine (B6)	6 mg
Cyanocobalamin (B12)	5 mcg
Biotin (H)	60 mcg
Folic acid	600 mcg
Ascorbic acid (C)	200 mg
Dose	10 mL/day (added daily to PN)

Table 7. Metabolic Functions of Vitamins

Vitamin	Metabolic functions
Fat-soluble vitamins	
Retinol (A)	Vision (rhodopsin: light-sensitive pigment), growth, reproduction
Calciferol (D3)	Calcium and phosphorus homeostasis
Tocopherol (E)	Antioxidant
Phytonadione (K1)	Synthesis of blood clotting factors II, VII, IX, X
Water-soluble vitamins	
Thiamine (B1)	Coenzyme in oxidative decarboxylation and transketolase enzyme
Riboflavin (B2)	Active coenzymes for oxidative reactions requiring electron transport
Niacin (B3)	Essential components of coenzymes (e.g., nicotinamide adenine dinucleotide; nicotinamide adenine dinucleotide phosphate); assist in oxidation-reduction reactions
Pantothenic acid (B5)	Constituent of coenzyme A necessary for acyl transfers; essential for energy production from metabolism of protein, carbohydrates, and fat
Pyridoxine (B6)	Pyridoxal phosphate is coenzyme involved in metabolic transformations of amino acids (decarboxylation, transamination, racemization), essential for neurotransmitter synthesis; required for heme synthesis
Cyanocobalamin (B12)	Coenzyme for DNA synthesis; involved in protein, carbohydrate, and lipid metabolism; conversion of homocysteine to methionine; essential for nervous system functioning
Biotin (H)	Cofactor for carboxylation reactions (e.g., carboxylation of Acetyl-CoA in fatty acid synthesis; carboxylation of pyruvate in gluconeogenesis) that are important in protein, carbohydrate, fatty acids, and nucleic acid metabolism
Folic acid	Transport of single carbon units, coenzyme in nucleic acid synthesis and metabolism of some amino acids
Ascorbic acid (C)	Antioxidant, cofactor in hydroxylation reactions and regulation of intracellular oxidation-reduction potentials, role in certain neurotransmitter and vasoactive amine synthesis, collagen synthesis

TRACE ELEMENTS

Trace elements are essential for normal metabolism, are normally abundant in the human body, and are physiologically required in relatively small amounts. During stress, tissue trace element redistribution occurs, which may lead to low serum trace element concentrations without necessarily indicating trace element deficiencies. Parenteral multi-trace element formulations usually contain zinc, copper, manganese, chromium, and selenium. Deficiencies or accumulation of trace elements may occur in the setting of disease states or abnormal trace element supplementation or accumulation. Clinical studies of patients treated with continuous renal replacement therapy (CRRT) showed clinically insignificant trace element losses across the hemodiafilter. Appendix A provides information on trace element deficiencies, toxicities, monitoring, and supplementation. Regular monitoring of trace element status (e.g., every 3 to 6 months) is recommended especially during long-term PN therapy. Table 8 provides the content of the adult multiple trace elements injection formulation (Multitrace[®]-5-Concentrate) available on Formulary.

Parenteral trace element formulations and supplementation are based on the 1988 recommendations for daily intravenous supplements of trace elements in the absence of deficiencies by the Nutrition Advisory Group of American Medical Association and the Society of Clinical Nutrition. These recommendations were questioned by the Safe Practice Guidelines by the American Society for Parenteral and Enteral Nutrition (A.S.P.E.N.) that published different guidelines for daily parenteral trace element requirements and supplementation (Table 9). Table 10 describes the known metabolic functions of trace elements.

Table 8. Composition and Dosing of Multitrace[®] 5-Concentrate in Adults

Multitrace[®] 5-Concentrate	Zinc (sulfate)	Copper (sulfate)	Manganese (sulfate)	Chromium (chloride)	Selenium (selenious acid)
1 mL	5 mg	1 mg	0.5 mg	10 mcg	60 mcg
Dose: 1 mL/day of Multitrace[®] 5-Concentrate is added to daily PN[a]					

[a]Unless otherwise indicated.

Table 9. Daily Parenteral Trace Element Requirements in Parenteral Nutrition for Adults and Adolescents According to A.S.P.E.N. Guidelines

Age Group	Zinc	Copper	Manganese	Chromium	Selenium
Adults (mg/day)	2.5–5	0.3–0.5	0.06–0.1	0.01–0.015	0.02–0.06
Adolescents > 40 Kg (mg/day)	2–5	0.2–0.5	0.04–0.1	0.005– 0.015	0.04–0.06

Single parenteral trace elements are available on Formulary and can be used as supplements to meet individual trace element requirements:

Chromium (chloride)	4 mcg/mL
Copper (chloride)	0.4 mg/mL
Manganese (sulfate)	0.1 mg/mL
Molybdenum (ammonium)	25 mcg/mL
Selenium (selenious acid)	40 mcg/mL
Zinc (chloride)	1 mg/mL

Table 10. Metabolic Functions and Serum Levels of Trace Elements

Trace element	Metabolic functions	Serum Levels
Zinc	Metabolism of proteins, lipids, carbohydrates, nucleic acids	0.55–1.5 mcg/mL
Selenium	Cofactor for glutathione peroxidase	Varies with age[a]
Copper	Associated with oxidative enzymes, collagen synthesis, iron metabolism	Males: 0.7–1.4 µg/mL Females: 0.7–1.6 µg/mL
Manganese	Associated with mucopolysaccharide metabolism, oxidative phosphorylation	0.40–0.85 ng/mL
Chromium	Potentiation of insulin effects through the glucose tolerance factor	< 0.3 ng/mL

[a]Age 0–2 months: 45–90 ng/mL; age 3–6 months: 50–120 ng/mL; age 7–9 months: 60–120 ng/mL; age 10–12 months: 70–130 ng/mL; age 1–10 years: 70–150 ng/mL; age 11–150 years: 95–165 ng/mL.

Zinc

Zinc is primarily eliminated via the intestines. Renal excretion usually accounts for a small fraction of zinc excretion, with normally up to 95% of renally excreted zinc being reabsorbed in the distal tubules. Although patients with high output ileostomy fluid losses or protracted diarrhea may lose up to 12 to 17 mg/L of small bowel fluid losses, zinc supplementation at 15 mg/day (elemental zinc) would likely maintain normal serum zinc concentrations in these patients. Significant fecal zinc losses also occur in patients with short bowel syndrome, and enterocutaneous fistulae.

Selenium

Selenium is primarily excreted via the kidneys. Significant selenium losses occur through the feces in patients with short bowel syndrome, high output ileostomy, and enterocutaneous fistulae. Under these conditions, higher selenium supplementation may be required at about 90 to 150 mcg/day to correct or maintain normal serum selenium concentrations.

Chromium

Chromium is primarily excreted via the kidneys. Because chromium is a contaminant of products used in the making of PN admixtures, additional chromium supplementation in PN formulations may not be necessary in long-term PN patients. Chromium supplementation should be guided by regular monitoring of serum chromium concentrations.

Copper

Copper is primarily eliminated via the bile. Patients with severe chronic cholestasis may have copper accumulation that necessitates copper restriction in PN.

Manganese

Manganese is mostly eliminated via the bile. Patients with cholestasis accumulate manganese, which may result in neurotoxicity. Manganese restriction is indicated in patients with cholestasis (Chapter XII).

MEDICATION ADDITIVES TO THE PARENTERAL NUTRIITON ADMIXTURE

Histamine-2 Receptor Antagonists

Histamine-2 receptor antagonists (H_2RAs) are compatible with PN admixtures. H_2RAs can be added to PN admixtures for stress ulcer prophylaxis, or to treat gastric hypersecretory conditions while the patient is receiving PN. The entire 24-hour dose can be added to the PN admixture on a daily basis (Table 11). Some advantages of continuous infusion of H_2RA over intermittent bolus doses include continuous control of gastric pH and saving nursing time.

Table 11. Daily Intravenous Histamine-2 Receptor Antagonists Dosing in PN for Adults[a]

H_2RA	Usual Daily Dose	Cl_{Cr}[b] 10–50 mL/min	Cl_{Cr}[b] < 10 mL/min
Ranitidine	150 mg[c]	100 mg	50 mg

[a]Doses vary depending on indication and clinical condition treated.
[b]Cl_{Cr} = creatinine clearance.

Estimated Cl_{Cr} (mL/min) for adults ($\geq$ 18 years of age):

Male= $\dfrac{(140 - age) \times weight\ (kg)}{72 \times Serum\ creatinine}$ 　　Female= Cl_{Cr} (male) x 0.85

[c]Maximum ranitidine dose is 300 mg per PN bag per day for adult patients.

Regular Human Insulin

Regular human insulin may be added to the PN admixture when hyperglycemia persists despite slow PN initiation and absence of dextrose overfeeding. Serum glucose concentrations are best to be maintained within a reasonable target range of 110 to 150 mg/dL. The minimum regular insulin dose to be added to the PN admixture for adult patients is 10 units per PN bag, because up to 40% of the insulin dose may adsorb to the PN bag and intravenous tubing. Maximum regular insulin in PN should not exceed 100 units/L of PN admixture. If a higher insulin dose is required, a continuous regular insulin infusion should be initiated to allow better titration of the insulin dose. When a continuous insulin infusion or sliding scale regular insulin regimen is used, about 70% of the previous day's insulin dose can be added to the subsequent PN admixture. The insulin dose should be adjusted based on frequent laboratory or capillary glucose measurements. Typically, intravenous insulin requirements in the PN admixture, to maintain euglycemia in patients with diabetes, range from 0.05 to 0.2 unit of insulin for each gram of dextrose in the PN admixture. Lower insulin doses may be required in patients with acute kidney injury, chronic kidney disease, or severe liver disease due to decreased insulin metabolism and potential for insulin accumulation that may lead to hypoglycemia. Reductions to the insulin dose are necessary when metabolic stress decreases, pancreatitis resolves, and when corticosteroid doses are tapered or discontinued. Regular laboratory or capillary glucose measurements (e.g., every 4 to 6 hours) should be instituted when insulin is added to PN.

Parenteral Iron

Iron is not routinely added to PN and is not a component of the parenteral trace elements. Iron dextran may be added to the PN admixture for maintenance or replacement for iron deficiency. Iron deficiency anemia may occur in patients requiring long-term PN, especially in patients with malabsorption diseases (e.g., short bowel syndrome).

Only sodium chloride-containing iron products should be used intravenously. Phenol-containing iron products are for intramuscular use only. Iron dextran is the only parenteral iron product that can be added to the lipid-free PN. Iron dextran should only be used when the oral route is not feasible, intestinal iron absorption is unreliable, or with gastrointestinal intolerance to oral iron supplements. Iron dextran should not be mixed or co-infused with intravenous lipid emulsions, because iron causes intravenous lipid emulsions to "oil out." Administration of iron dextran in infected patients should be avoided due to concerns of increased bacterial proliferation, as bacteria may use iron for growth.

Immediate or delayed anaphylactic reactions have been reported with and following the administration of iron injection. Severe reactions may occur during or following iron dextran administration and may include fever, chills, backache, myalgia, dizziness, syncope, and rash. Severe hypersensitivity reactions characterized by cardiovascular collapse, cardiac arrest, bronchospasm, dyspnea, angioedema, urticaria, and muscle spasm have been reported with parenteral iron therapy.

Prior to iron dextran administration, a test dose must be given to determine the patient's susceptibility. In adults, an iron dextran test dose of 25 mg (0.5 mL) may be diluted in 25 to 50 mL of 0.9% sodium chloride and administered over 15 minutes. Patients should be observed closely for hypersensitivity reactions for one hour before the remainder of the initial dose is administered.

For iron deficiency not due to blood loss, the total replacement dosage (mg of elemental iron) is calculated as follows:

$$\text{Total iron (mg)} = 0.66 \times \text{body weight (kg)} \times \left[100 - \frac{\text{hemoglobin (g/dL)} \times 100}{14.8}\right]$$

Up to 100 mg of iron dextran may be added daily to PN (not containing intravenous lipid emulsions) until the total replacement iron dose is administered. Alternatively, the total iron dose may be diluted in 250 to 1000 mL of 0.9% sodium chloride and infused over 4 to 6 hours.

Other parenteral iron formulations including iron sucrose and sodium ferric gluconate should not be added or co-infused with PN admixtures. Iron sucrose and sodium ferric gluconate have been associated with lower rate of serious hypersensitivity reactions compared to iron dextran, have been safely administered to patients with documented hypersensitivity reactions with iron dextran, and do not usually require a test dose.

MEDICATIONS COMPATIBILITY WITH PARENTERAL NUTRITION ADMIXTURES

Several factors influence the chemical and physical stability and compatibility of intravenous admixtures. These include pH, concentrations, temperature, order of mixing, and time after mixing. Limitations to the medication-PN compatibility data include:
- Lack of compatibility data with every PN component.
- Compatibility studies are mostly based on visual assessment rather chemical analysis.
- Compatibility data with intravenous lipid emulsions are limited. Intravenous lipid emulsions are easily destabilized especially in an acidic milieu, and the opaque color of lipids may mask visualization of any precipitates. Further, lipid particles carry negative charges on their external surface that can be disrupted by divalent or trivalent cations

(*zeta* potential). When necessary, intravenous lipid emulsion infusions can be interrupted to infuse medications.

Medications that can be added to mixed protein and dextrose PN include intravenous vitamins, electrolytes, trace elements, heparin (low dose), insulin, and histamine-2 receptor antagonists.

Human albumin is a plasma volume expander, has no nutritional value, and should not be used for nutritional purpose. Adding albumin to PN admixture is not advised because albumin may increase the potential for microbial growth in PN admixtures.

Hydrochloric acid (HCl) has bee reportedly added to PN admixtures (maximum of 100 mEq/L of 0.1N HCl) to correct severe metabolic alkalosis. However, HCl is incompatible with intravenous lipid emulsions, and it is recommended that HCl be administered in a separate intravenous infusion because acidosis may develop quickly. Frequent and close monitoring of blood pH and serum electrolytes is required with HCl infusion.

Medication compatibility with PN admixtures should first be confirmed before an intravenous medication is added or co-infused with a PN admixture. Refer to Appendix K for compatibility information on medication infused with PN using a "Y" connector tubing site. For more medication compatibility information with PN admixtures, contact the Drug Information Service (phone 734-936-8200) during work hours or the 24-hour open satellite inpatient Pharmacies (Mott Hospital phone 734-764-8208; Main Hospital 6th floor satellite phone 734-936-8251).

TRANSITION FROM PARENTERAL TO ENTERAL NUTRITION OR ORAL DIET

EN should be initiated prior to the discontinuation of PN therapy. PN should be decreased as EN is advanced and tolerated. Transition from PN to EN should be monitored to ensure that patients continue to receive their nutritional requirements during transition. PN is discontinued once enteral feeding is tolerated at approximately 75% of the desired nutritional goal.

For patients transitioning to oral diet, ordering two- or three-day calorie counts during transition off PN allows quantification of calorie and protein intake from oral diet (or supplements). Once approximately 75% of the estimated nutritional requirements are taken orally, PN is tapered off and discontinued. Chapter V provides information on EN for adults and adolescents. Appendix B shows a list of available adult EN formulas available on Formulary.

VII. MONITORING NUTRITION SUPPORT THERAPY FOR ADULT PATIENTS

After the initial nutrition assessment and followed by the initiation of nutrition support therapy, the patient's response to nutrition support is evaluated by serial assessments of parameters such as body weight changes, serum visceral protein concentrations, nitrogen balance, wound healing, and other laboratory and physical parameters.

WEIGHT GAIN

If weight gain is the goal, an increase in body weight at an average of 0.1 to 0.2 kg/day is expected in adult patients receiving adequate nutrition support. Greater daily weight gain may suggest accumulation of excess fluid or fat.

VISCERAL PROTEINS

Serum visceral proteins (albumin, prealbumin, transferrin, retinol-binding protein) are used as markers of nutritional status. The interpretation of serum visceral protein concentrations in acute care patients is limited by their sensitivity and specificity. Albumin, prealbumin, transferrin, and retinol-binding protein are "negative" acute phase proteins. Their serum concentrations are reduced in response to stress or injury (e.g., severe trauma, thermal injury, sepsis, surgery, organ failure) in the absence of malnutrition. Other conditions that may also affect visceral proteins are shown in Table 1. Therefore, serum visceral protein concentrations should be interpreted by considering many factors including nutritional history, nutrition support therapy, concurrent and underlying diseases, and medication therapy.

The frequency of monitoring serum visceral protein concentrations is dictated by their respective half-lives. Because serum prealbumin has a shorter (~ $1/10^{th}$) half-life (~ 2 days) compared to albumin (~ 20 days), serum prealbumin concentrations provide a faster indication of protein body stores in response to nutrition support therapy. When used as a nutritional marker, serum prealbumin concentrations are monitored once weekly, and trended over time to assess progression and response to nutrition support therapy. Acute decrease in serum prealbumin concentrations, while a patient is receiving adequate nutrition, should be interpreted in light of the other factors that may have caused the change (particularly patient's intravascular volume), rather than solely as a function of the patient's nutritional status or inadequacy of nutrition support therapy. Serum prealbumin concentrations are influenced by protein and calorie intake. Providing adequate calories (along with adequate protein intake) especially from dextrose (in case of PN) spares proteins from being used for energy, and this will be reflected in improved serum prealbumin concentrations.

Table 1. Specificity and Sensitivity of Visceral Proteins to Assess Nutritional Status[a]

Serum protein	Half-life	Factors causing increased values	Factors causing decreased values	Advantages	Disadvantages
Albumin	~20 days	Dehydration Anabolic steroids Insulin	Overhydration Edema Renal insufficiency Nephrotic syndrome Trauma Thermal injury CHF Cirrhosis	Easily measured Prognostic index of clinical outcome	Large body pool Slow response to nutrition support Sensitive to non-nutritional factors
Prealbumin	~2-3 days	Renal dysfunction Steroids	Cirrhosis Hepatitis Inflammation Trauma Thermal injury	Smaller body pool Responds quickly to nutritional changes	Levels Affected by protein and caloric intake Sensitive to non-nutritional factors
Transferrin	8-10 days	Iron deficiency Pregnancy Chronic blood loss Hypoxia Estrogens	Chronic infection Cirrhosis Iron overdose Enteropathies Nephrotic syndrome Thermal injury Testosterone Steroids	Smaller body pool Responds quickly to nutritional changes	When calculated from TIBC, it is not as accurate as direct measurement
Retinol-binding protein	~12 hours	Renal dysfunction Vitamin A supplements	Same as prealbumin Vitamin A deficiency	Shortest half-life Sensitive to nutritional changes	Sensitive to non-nutritional factors

CHF = congestive heart failure; TIBC = total iron binding capacity.

NITROGEN BALANCE

Most body nitrogen is a component of proteins. Nitrogen is released during protein catabolism and is mainly excreted as urea in the urine. Nitrogen balance is the difference between body nitrogen gains and losses, and is the generally accepted method to evaluate the adequacy of protein intake and retention. It is based on the premise that nitrogen equilibrium is attained when the protein supply is adequate to replace losses via protein metabolism (mostly urea) and direct losses (in stools, urine, wounds, desquamation of epithelial cells, sweat). Protein synthesis depends in part on the patient's activity level. Physical exercise is essential for adequate regeneration of skeletal muscle, and patient's physical therapy should be emphasized. Nitrogen balance is calculated as follows:

Nitrogen balance (g/day) = nitrogen intake (g/day) – nitrogen losses (g/day)

Nitrogen accounts for about 16% (assuming protein is comprised of 16% nitrogen: 1/6.25 = 0.16) of protein structure. Nitrogen equivalent to protein is calculated as follows:

$$\text{Nitrogen intake} = \frac{\text{grams of protein intake from all sources}}{6.25}$$

Nitrogen losses are determined by measuring the excretion or accumulation of nitrogenous metabolic end products, particularly urea. In non-stressed patients, urinary urea nitrogen (UUN, in g/24 hours) accounts for about 80% to 90% of total urinary nitrogen (TUN). This estimation becomes invalid in critically ill patients and those with acute kidney injury, sepsis, and liver failure, whereby non-urea urinary nitrogen components vary with formation of non-urea nitrogen substances (e.g., ammonia, uric acid). Although TUN is a more accurate measurement than UUN, measuring TUN is laborious, and clinicians rely more on measuring UUN.

Nitrogen losses = UUN + non-urea urinary nitrogen (2 g) + fecal nitrogen (2 g)

Protein and calorie intake both affect nitrogen retention. A positive nitrogen balance reflects that nitrogen intake exceeds nitrogen loss. A desired positive nitrogen balance for the unstressed patient is in the range of 4 to 6 g/day. In a patient receiving nutrition support therapy, it is desirable to maintain at least a neutral or at best a positive nitrogen balance daily, realizing that the anabolic effects on protein synthesis may not be apparent for several days. Nitrogen balance should best be measured when a steady state of the clinical and nutritional aspects is achieved. A positive nitrogen balance is often difficult to achieve in critically ill patients unless the patient's stress level decreases. Further, nitrogen balance results may represent the degree of catabolism in critically ill catabolic patients rather than an indication of nutrition support adequacy. Also, a relationship between a positive nitrogen balance and patient outcomes has not been demonstrated.

OTHER MONITORING PARAMETERS

Table 2. Laboratory Monitoring of Nutrition Support Therapy in Hospitalized Patients[a]

	Initial	Daily (unstable)	1-2 times per week (stable)	As indicated
BUN, Creatinine, Glucose	X	X	X	
Na, K, Cl, CO_2, Mg, Ca, P	X	X	X	
AST, ALT, LDH, Alkaline Phosphatase, Bilirubin	X		X	X
GGT				X
Albumin	X		X	
Prealbumin				X
Triglycerides	X[b]		X	X
Hgb, Hct, CBC, Platelets, PT, PTT				X
Trace elements, Vitamins				X
TIBC, Ferritin				X

[a]Frequency of monitoring varies with clinical conditions. Critically ill patients or those with metabolic complications require more frequent laboratory monitoring.
[b]Measured once goal lipid infusion reached.

Table 3. Other Monitoring Parameters of Nutrition Support Therapy in Hospitalized Patients

	Every 8 hours	Daily	As indicated
Volume of intravenous infusions	X		
Oral intake	X		
Urine, Ostomy, Fistula, Nasogastric losses	X		
Body weight		X	
Body temperature	X		
Resting energy expenditure (REE)[a]			X
Urine glucose			X
Urine electrolytes			X
Urine urea nitrogen (UUN)			X

[a]Indirect calorimetry

ENTERAL NUTRITION MONITORITNG

Most complications related to the administration of EN can be easily treated and prevented through proper monitoring. During enteral feeding administration, the patient should be monitored for nausea, diarrhea, abdominal cramping, and bloating (Chapters VII and XI). Suggested EN monitoring guidelines are shown in Table 4.

Table 4. Other Monitoring Parameters for Patients Receiving Enteral Nutrition

	Initial	Daily	As indicated
Chemsticks			X
Intake and output	X	X	
Weight	X	X	
Feeding tube position and tube site [a]	X		X
Gastric residual volume [b]	X		X
Number and consistency of stools		X	
Abdominal distension		X	

[a] Check mark on tube, which denotes the exit point from the nares at the time of initial placement, or measure the length of tube exiting from the nares. Check tube position every 4 hours for continuous feeding or before each intermittent feeding. Notify physician if tube migration is suspected.

[b] Document reason(s) for interruption in tube feeding schedule such as procedures, high gastric residual volumes (GRV), clogged feeding tube. For gastric feeding, check GRV every 4 hours or prior to each intermittent feeding. Hold enteral feeding if GRV are greater than twice the hourly rate, and over 150 mL for intermittent feedings. Recheck GRV after 1 hour.

VIII. NUTRITION ASSESSMENT AND NUTRITIONAL REQUIREMENTS FOR PEDIATRIC PATIENTS

The pediatric population encompasses a wide range of individuals ranging from birth to 18 years of age. Pediatric nutrition assessment differs from that of adults due to growth requirements of pediatric patients. Therefore, the assessment of the pediatric patient's nutritional status is a principal step in designing an EN or PN support therapy. Prevention and treatment of malnutrition are especially important during childhood because of the negative consequences of inadequate calorie and protein intake on the child's growth and development.

EVALUATION OF NUTRITIONAL STATUS

It is essential to perform a subjective global assessment (SGA) with physical examination of the pediatric patient to evaluate the patient's nutritional status (refer to Chapter III for SGA description). The assessment of nutritional status includes a review of the diet history, medical history, physical examination, growth patterns, anthropometric measurements, and biochemical assessment. A detailed diet history is essential to assess the nutritional status. The feeding history of the child that is best obtained from the parent or caregiver should include the patient's first food as an infant, any foods that are excluded from the diet, and the reason and length of time of the dietary exclusion(s). Also, current intake and daily feeding schedules should be evaluated. Because certain medications may cause nutritional deficiencies, drug-nutrient interactions need to be considered in the evaluation of nutritional status.

Vitamin and mineral deficiencies are frequently associated with malnutrition. Although classic advanced signs and symptoms are occasionally encountered, stigmata of vitamin deficiencies are often mild and nonspecific, and may be confused with signs of non-nutritional abnormalities. Therefore, physical findings of malnutrition must be interpreted in light of the patient's history and anthropometric data. Chapter III provides information on the classic physical findings that suggest vitamin, mineral, and protein-energy deficiencies.

Monitoring the child's growth through serial measurements of weight, length or height, and head circumference is essential in determining the child's own growth curve. These measurements are plotted on the National Center for Health Statistics Centers for Disease Control and Prevention (NCHS/CDC) growth charts to evaluate the adequacy of physical growth. Growth charts are available in CareWeb under the "Continuity" tab. The NCHS/CDC growth charts can also be accessed on the following website: www.cdc.gov/growthcharts/. Special growth charts are also available for monitoring the growth of children with special health-care needs (e.g., Down syndrome, myelomeningocele, achondroplasia, Prader-Willi syndrome, cerebral palsy, etc.).

ESTIMATION OF NUTRITIONAL REQUIREMENTS

Dietary Reference Intakes

Historically, the Recommended Dietary Allowances (RDAs) were used to calculate energy requirements for pediatric patients (Appendix L). The RDAs have been replaced by the Dietary Reference Intakes (DRIs). The DRIs were developed by the Institute of Medicine, Food, and Nutrition Board for the United States and Canada, and describe the "reference values that are quantitative estimates of nutrient intakes to be used for planning and assessing diets of healthy people." The DRIs include the Estimated Average Requirement (EAR, nutrient intake value estimated to meet the requirement of half the healthy individuals in an age- and gender-specific group), the Tolerable Upper Intake Level (UL, highest level of a daily nutrient intake that is likely to pose no risks of adverse health effects to almost all individuals in the group to whom it is designed), and the RDAs (average daily dietary intake level that is sufficient to meet the nutrient requirements of nearly all, 97% to 98%, healthy individuals in an age- and gender-specific group). The DRIs help individuals optimize health, prevent disease, avoid consuming too much of a nutrient, and can be used by health professionals to assess nutrient intake and plan diets for individuals and groups. For complete and updated listing of DRIs, visit the Institute of Medicine website at: http://www.iom.edu/.

Energy Requirements

DRIs for energy requirements and appropriate growth for healthy children and adolescents with a body mass index (BMI) of 18.5 to 25 kg/m^2 are shown in Table 1. Other specific energy requirements are shown in Tables 2, 3, 4, and 5.

Protein Requirements

For most term infants with normal kidney and liver functions, protein intake at 2.5 g/kg/day achieves positive nitrogen balance. Daily protein requirements for pediatric patients are shown in Table 6.

Table 1. Estimated Daily Energy Requirements for Children and Adolescents based on Dietary Reference Intakes

Age	Energy requirements (kcal/day)
Infants and Young Children (months)	
0–3	(89 x W – 100) + 175
4–6	(89 x W – 100) + 56
7–12	(89 x W – 100) + 22
13–35	(89 x W – 100) + 20
Children and Adolescents Boys (years)	
3–8 years	88.5 – (61.9 x A) + PA x (26.7 x W) + (903 x H) + 20
9–18 years	88.5 – (61.9 x A) + PA x (26.7 x W) + (903 x H) + 25
Children and Adolescents Girls (years)	
3–8 years	135.3 – (30.8 x A) + PA x (10 x W) + (934 x H) + 20
9–18 years	135.3 – (30.8 x A) + PA x (10 x W) + (934 x H) + 25
Activity Level	
Sedentary	TDL: Boys 1; Girls 1
Low active	TDL + 30 to 60" daily moderate activity: Boys 1.13; Girls 1.16
Active	TDL + > 60" daily moderate activity: Boys 1.26; Girls 1.31
Very active	TDL + > 120" daily moderate activity or 60" moderate + 60" vigorous activity: Boys 1.42; Girls 1.56

W = weight (kg); A = age (years); H = height (m); PA = Physical Activity Coefficient; TDL = typical daily living.
From: Food and Nutrition Board, Institute of Medicine, National Academy of Sciences. Dietary Reference Intakes: Recommended Intakes for Individuals; 2006.

When indirect calorimetry is not available for use in critically ill patients on ventilator support, predictive equations are used to determine energy requirements. Energy requirements for pediatric patients with chronic illnesses are shown in Table 2. The World Health Organization (WHO) equations to estimate the resting energy expenditure (REE) are shown in Table 3. The Schofield predictive equations for energy requirements, used for children and adolescents, are shown in Table 4. Parenteral energy requirements are shown in Table 5, and are lower than enteral requirements due to less thermogenesis and absence of energy loss in stools.

Table 2. Estimated Energy Requirements for Pediatric Patients Based on Chronic Health Conditions

Medical diagnosis	Energy calculation estimate

Down syndrome	Children 5–11 year of age:
	  Girls 14.3 kcal/cm
	  Boys 16.1 kcal/cm

Spina bifida	Children over 8 years of age and minimally active:
	Weight maintenance: 9–11 kcal/cm, or 50%
	  fewer calories than recommended for a child
	  of the same age without the condition
	Weight loss: 7 kcal/cm

Prader-Willi syndrome	All children and adolescents:
	  Growth maintenance: 10–11 kcal/cm
	  Slow weight loss/support linear growth: 8.5 kcal/cm

Children with very low energy requirements	Lower energy requirements: 7–9 kcal/cm Moderate energy requirements: 9–10 kcal/cm High energy requirements: 12–15 kcal/cm

From: Lucas BL, eds. Children with Special Health Care Needs, Nutrition Care Handbook. 1st ed. Chicago: American Dietetic Association; 2004.

Table 3. Resting Energy Expenditure Based on the World Health Organization Equations

Age (years)	Resting energy expenditure (kcal/day)	
0–3	Males	$(60.9 \times W) - 54$
	Females	$(61 \times W) - 51$
3–10	Males	$(22.7 \times W) + 495$
	Females	$(22.5 \times W) + 499$
10–18	Males	$(17.5 \times W) + 651$
	Females	$(12.2 \times W) + 746$

W = weight (kg).
From: World Health Organization. Energy and protein requirements. Report of a joint FAO/WHO/UNC Expert Consultation. Technical Report Series No. 724: Geneva: World Health Organization 1985;206.

Table 4. Resting Energy Expenditure Using the Schofield Equations[a]

Age (years)	Basal metabolic rate (kcal/day)	
< 3	Males	$(0.167 \times W) + (15.16 \times H) - 617.1$
	Females	$(16.24 \times W) + (10.22 \times H) - 413.2$
3–10	Males	$(19.58 \times W) + (1.3 \times H) + 414.6$
	Females	$(16.95 \times W) + (1.61 \times H) + 370.9$
10–18	Males	$(16.24 \times W) + (1.37 \times H) + 515.1$
	Females	$(8.35 \times W) + (4.65 \times H) + 199.9$

W = weight (kg); H = height (cm).
[a]The Schofield equations are reliable at predicting REE, especially in less than 10 year-old children.
From: Schofield WN. Predicting basal metabolic rate, new standards and review of previous work. Hum Nutr Clinic Nutr 1985;39(suppl 1):5-41.

Table 5. Estimated Energy Requirements in Parenteral Nutrition for Pediatric Patients

Age (years)	Energy requirements (kcal/kg/day)
Preterm	90–110
0–1	90–100
1–7	75–90
7–12	60–75
12–18	30–60

From: Koletzko B, Goulet O, Hunt J, et al. Parenteral Nutrition Guidelines Working Group; European Society for Clinical Nutrition and Metabolism; European Society of Paediatric Gastroenterology, Hepatology and Nutrition (ESPGHAN); European Society of Paediatric Research (ESPR). Guidelines on Paediatric Parenteral Nutrition of ESPGHAN and the European Society for Clinical Nutrition and Metabolism (ESPEN), supported by ESPR. J Pediatr Gastroenterol Nutr 2005;41(Suppl 2):S5-11.

Table 6. Daily Protein Requirements for Pediatric Patients[a]

Pediatric patient/birth weight	Protein requirements (g/kg/day)[a]
< 1000 g	3.5–3.8
1000–2500 g	3–3.5
Term neonate	2.5–3
Older children	1.5–2
Adolescents	1–1.5

[a]Protein requirements are adjusted based or underlying diseases, clinical conditions, nutritional status, and protein tolerance.

EVALUATION AND MONITORING OF NUTRITION SUPPORT

One of the most useful assessment parameters of nutritional status in the pediatric patient is growth. Anthropometric measurements of weight, length/height, and head circumference can be used to assess growth cross-sectionally or longitudinally. One-time measurements of any of these parameters can be compared to age-appropriate reference charts. Serial measurements are a good indicator for growth velocity and appropriateness of nutrition support therapy. Inadequate weight gain may suggest an underlying metabolic or clinical problem. Excessive weight gain may reflect excess fluid administration and retention. Expected weight gains in children are shown in Table 7. Calorie intake can be adjusted at time intervals based on periodic growth velocity measurements, as shown in Table 8. The classification of protein-energy malnutrition is shown in Table 9.

In addition to the NCHS growth charts, weight records of preterm infants should be closely monitored. Former preterm infants' anthropometric data should be corrected for appropriate gestational age when plotted on the NCHS growth charts until 2.5 years of age.

Serum visceral proteins are also used in nutritional assessment. Serum albumin and prealbumin concentrations are measured regularly to determine nutritional efficacy. Because protein-energy malnutrition may impair immune function and increase the patient's risk for infection, total lymphocyte count (TLC) has been used as a surrogate marker to assess immune function. Refer to Chapter IV for details on nutritional assessment.

Table 7. Expected Weight Gain Relative to Age for Children

Age	Weight gain (g/day)
0–3 months	25–35
Over 3–6 months	15–21
Over 6–12 months	10–13
Over 1–6 years	5–8
Over 6–10 years	5–11

Table 8. Minimal Time Intervals for Growth Velocity Measurements

Measurement	Interval
Weight	7 days
Length	4 weeks
Height	8 weeks
Head circumference	7 days (infants) 4 weeks (up to 3 years of age)

Table 9. Classification of Protein-Energy Malnutrition

Type of PEM[a]	Anthropometric index as % of standard[a]	Degree of protein-energy malnutrition			
		Normal	Mild	Moderate	Severe
Chronic (stunting)	Height for age	95	90–94	85–89	< 85
Acute (wasting)	Weight for age	90	75–89	60–74	< 60
	Weight for height	90	80–89	70–79	< 70

[a]The 50th percentile of the NCHS growth charts is the commonly used standard. Adapted with permission from: Bessler S. Nutritional assessment. In: Samour PQ, King K, eds. Handbook of Pediatric Nutrition. 3rd ed. Sudbury, MA: Jones and Bartlett Publishers, Inc;2005:11-33.

[a]The 50th percentile of the NCHS growth charts is the commonly used standard. Adapted with permission from: Bessler S. Nutritional assessment. In: Samour PQ, King K, eds. Handbook of Pediatric Nutrition. 3rd ed. Sudbury, MA: Jones and Bartlett Publishers, Inc;2005:11-33.

INTESTINAL FAILURE AND SURGICAL SHORT BOWEL SYNDROME

Intestinal failure is characterized by reduced capacity of the intestines to absorb adequate nutrients, water, and electrolytes to maintain proper health and growth. Patients may have normal intestinal length but have intestinal dysmotility, radiation enteritis, or malabsorption disorders that prevent adequate absorption. In children, intestinal loss, surgical resection, or injury, could result from necrotizing enterocolitis, midgut volvulus, abdominal wall defects, intestinal atresias, vascular infarct, cloacal extrophy, long segment Hirschsprung's disease, abdominal trauma, or severe inflammatory bowel disease.

Significant intestinal resection could result in short bowel syndrome. Short bowel syndrome can be defined as resection or functional loss of the small intestine, leaving less than 30% of the normal small intestine length-for-age in infants, and less than 200 cm in adults. This could result in malabsorption, disorders of fluids, electrolytes, and minerals, intestinal losses of vitamins and trace elements, malnutrition, and possible linear growth deficits in infants and children. Refer to Chapter III for sites of intestinal nutrients absorption (Figure 1) and the clinical physical characteristics of nutritional deficiencies (Table 1). Appendix A provides information on micronutrient deficiencies, toxicities, and replacement.

The management of intestinal failure and short bowel syndrome patients requires early intervention and long-term care. These patients require special nutritional management, whether with parenteral and/or enteral nutrition or with nutrient supplements. The University of Michigan Mott Children's Hospital, Department of Pediatrics and Pediatric Surgery Children's Intestinal Rehabilitation Program, provides interdisciplinary care to patients with intestinal failure and short bowel syndrome. For information on the University of Michigan CHIRP, visit the following public website: http://surgery.med.umich.edu/pediatric/sbs/.

IX. ENTERAL NUTRITION FOR PEDIATRIC PATIENTS

Enteral nutrition (EN) is indicated for pediatric patients with a functional gastrointestinal tract, who are unable to ingest sufficient nutrients by mouth to maintain health, growth, and development. Contraindications for EN for pediatrics patient include necrotizing enterocolitis, gastrointestinal obstruction, severe inflammatory bowel disease, and severe protracted diarrhea. Successful EN requires appropriate formula selection and feeding regimen.

ENTERAL NUTRITION FORMULA SELECTION

Only infant formulas are regulated by the Food and Drug Administration (FDA) and are under the category of "foods for special dietary use" (Infant Formula Act of 1980). All other EN formulas are considered "medical foods" and are not regulated by the FDA. Therefore, they are exempt from labeling and health-claim regulations such as those that apply to drugs.

The different categories of pediatric EN formulas are based on the relative maturity of the child's gastrointestinal tract, liver, kidneys, and age-specific nutrient requirements. These categories include EN formulas for preterm infants; full-term infants less than 1 year of age; children 1 to 10 years of age; and children with inborn errors of metabolism.

Infant and pediatric oral nutrient and EN feeding formulas available on Formulary are shown in Appendix N, and updates are shown on the Patient Food and Nutrition Services internal website: http://www.med.umich.edu/i/pfans.

HUMAN MILK

Human milk is recommended as the main nutrition source for the first 4 to 6 months of age. The American Academy of Pediatrics (AAP) recommends that breastfeeding continues for at least one year of age. Human milk is a rich source of nutrients and non-nutritional bioactive components needed by the neonate as it contains antimicrobial factors, cytokines, anti-inflammatory substances, hormones, growth modulators, and digestive enzymes. Human milk composition varies among individuals, with the stage of lactation, breastfeeding pattern, and parity. The caloric density of human milk is approximately 20 kcal/oz.

Reports of vitamin D deficiency and rickets in breastfed infants led the AAP to recommend supplemental vitamin D 400 IU per day for all breastfed and non-breastfed infants who do not receive at least 1000 mL of daily vitamin D-fortified formula or milk, beginning within the first few days of life. This can be provided with a daily multivitamin supplement containing the required vitamin

D amounts. Because human milk may contain insufficient amounts of protein, calcium, phosphorus, and sodium to meet the nutritional requirements of the preterm infant, human milk fortifiers are added to the human milk given to preterm infants. For most infants, foods should be introduced after 4 to 6 months of age when nutrient intake from human milk may become insufficient.

PREMATURE INFANT FORMULAS

Premature infant formulas are designed for infants who weigh less than 2500 g. Ready-to-feed formulas are available in concentrations of 20, 24, and 30 kcal/oz. Similac Special Care® 30 may be added to a base of 24 kcal/oz premie feeds to make 26, 27, or 28 kcal/oz premie feeds. Similac Special Care® and Enfamil Premature LIPIL® are available with low-iron (0.37 to 0.5 mg/100 kcal) and standard iron-fortified (1.8 mg/100 kcal) formulas. Low-iron formulas should not be used in patients with or at risk for iron deficiency anemia. Preterm infants may not tolerate feeding formulas with increased caloric densities that could potentially lead to feeding intolerance or necrotizing enterocolitis. When feeding volume cannot be advanced and additional nutrients are required for growth, caloric density of formulas should be gradually increased with monitoring for gastrointestinal tolerance and hydration status. The final osmolarity of the feeding formula should not exceed 400 mOsm/L (osmolality less than 450 mOsm/kg of water).

Sources of carbohydrate, protein, and fat in premature infant formulas are tailored to meet the unique requirements of this age group. They contain glucose polymers that decrease the lactose load to the premature infant for ease of digestion. They have higher protein concentrations and the digestibility of proteins is improved with a whey-to-casein ratio of 60-to-40. Whey proteins form smaller curds and are more easily digested than casein. These formulas contain a higher percentage of medium-chain triglycerides (MCT) that are useful to improve fat absorption in preterm infants with reduced bile acids pool who have difficulty absorbing long-chain fatty acids. Premature infant formulas have higher calcium and phosphorus compared to term infant formulas, because of the higher demand for calcium and phosphate for bone and skeletal growth in preterm infants.

TRANSITIONAL FORMULAS

Transitional EN formulas are intended for preterm infants at the time of hospital discharge, and can be used in infants through one year of corrected gestational age. Transitional formulas provide nutrient composition in between that of a concentrated premature and a term infant formula. These formulas also have higher protein, MCT, vitamin, and mineral content compared to standard infant formulas. Ready-to-feed transitional formulas available on Formulary are Similac Neosure® and Enfamil Enfacare Lipil® with a caloric density of 22 kcal/oz.

TERM INFANT FORMULAS

Cow Milk-Based Formulas

The formulas of choice for full-term infants who are not breastfed and do not have underlying gastrointestinal disorders are cow milk-based iron-fortified formulas that have nutrient composition that closely approximates human milk. These formulas are available in standard dilutions at concentrations of 20 kcal/oz (0.67 kcal/mL). Formulas can be made more concentrated up to 30 kcal/oz (1 kcal/mL), when medically indicated (e.g., infants with fluid restriction or with increased metabolic needs). When high-formula concentrations are used, feeding tolerance, hydration status, fluid and electrolyte balance, and renal function should be closely monitored. Cow milk-based formulas available on Formulary include Enfamil LIPIL®, Similac Advance Early Shield®, and Carnation Good Start Supreme®. These term infant formulas contain arachidonic acid (ARA) and docosahexaenoic acid (DHA), which are fatty acids found naturally in human milk and are believed to be essential for brain and eye development. To help strengthen the immune system, Similac Advance Early Shield® also contains a prebiotic, nucleotides, and antioxidants in a combination similar to human milk. In patients with galactosemia, a lactose-free formula such as Enfamil Lactofree LIPIL® can be used.

Soy-Based Formulas

Soy-based formulas are lactose-free term infant formulas that contain soy protein isolates as the protein source. They are available in 20 kcal/oz (0.67 kcal/mL) concentration, but can be made more concentrated. They are indicated for use in infants with galactosemia, hereditary lactase deficiency, and as a "vegetarian diet." They are contraindicated in infants with sucrase-isomaltase deficiency and hereditary fructose intolerance. They should not be used in infants who have milk-protein allergy or intolerance because about one-third of children with adverse reactions to milk-based formulas also react to soy. Soy formulas are not designed or recommended for use in preterm infants because they contain high aluminum concentrations that may cause osteopenia. Further, infants who were fed soy formulas had low serum phosphorus and high serum alkaline phosphatase concentrations associated with the development of osteopenia. Examples of soy-based formulas available on Formulary are Enfamil Prosobee LIPIL®, Similac Isomil Advance®, and Carnation Good Start Supreme Soy®.

Modified Fat Source Formulas

Modified fat source high MCT lactose-free formulas are indicated in patients with severe fat malabsorption, steatorrhea, or chylothorax. Pregestimil LIPIL®, which is made with protein hydrolysates and contains 55% of the fat source as MCT, can be used in infants with liver disease, cholestasis, cystic fibrosis, and other malabsorption syndromes such as short bowel syndrome and pancreatic insufficiency. Portagen® contains up to 85% of its fat source as MCT, and is used in patients with chylothorax. Because high MCT-based formulas are low in long-chain fatty acids, patients should be monitored for signs of essential fatty acid deficiency (Chapter XII) when these formulas are used as the sole source of nutrition and fat intake for extended periods.

Semi-Elemental Formulas

Semi-elemental or protein hydrolysate formulas are hypoallergenic, lactose-free, and contain hydrolyzed casein. Some semi-elemental formulas also contain MCT. These formulas are mainly used for patients with food allergies, cow's milk protein allergy, soy protein allergy, inflammatory bowel disease, colic due to protein sensitivity, and intractable diarrhea. Examples of protein hydrolysate formulas are Pregestimil LIPIL®, Similac Alimentum®, and Nutramigen LIPIL® that does not contain MCT.

Elemental Formulas

Elemental or amino-acid formulas have their protein source digested in the form of free amino acids. They do not contain milk or soy protein, lactose, galactose, fructose, or gluten, and are relatively low in their fat content. Elemental formulas are appropriate for pediatric patients with malabsorption (e.g., short bowel syndrome, intestinal fistulae, eosinophilic gastrointestinal disorders), and for infants with severe protein intolerance and food allergy who poorly respond to semi-elemental formulas. Examples include EleCare® and Neocate®.

Low Mineral Content Formula

Infants with impaired kidney function may require a low mineral content formula such as Similac PM 60/40®, a cow milk-based formula with a whey-to-casein ratio of 60-to-40. Similac PM 60/40® provides minerals at levels closely approximating human milk with a calcium-to-phosphate ratio of 2-to-1 that is designed to help treat calcium and phosphate disorders. It is a low-iron (0.7 mg/100 kcal) formula and additional iron supplementation from other sources is necessary. Additional electrolyte supplementation may also be needed when Similac PM 60/40® is used in patients with gastrointestinal or urinary mineral and electrolyte losses.

ENTERAL FORMULAS FOR CHILDREN ONE to TEN YEARS OF AGE

Cow Milk-Based Formulas

Cow milk-based intact protein formulas with a caloric density of 1 kcal/mL are available for children 1 to 10 years of age who are nutritionally depleted but are otherwise healthy. Cow milk-based intact protein formulas are lactose-free and contain age-appropriate amounts of vitamins and minerals. Examples of cow milk-based formulas are Nutren Jr® and PediaSure®. Fiber-supplemented formula such as Nutren Jr with fiber® can be used to help regulate bowel motility in patients with constipation or diarrhea. Resource Just for Kids 1.5 Cal® (with or without fiber) is a high-calorie (1.5 kcal/mL) formula for children who have increased calorie requirements, but have fluid restrictions or do not tolerate high gastric feeding volumes.

Semi-Elemental and Elemental Formulas

Semi-elemental and elemental EN formulas are lactose-free, contain MCT oil, and have a caloric density of 0.8 to 1 kcal/mL. These formulas are indicated in pediatric patients with malabsorption (e.g., short bowel syndrome, intestinal fistula). Peptamen Junior® is a semi-elemental formula with enzymatically hydrolyzed whey protein. Examples of elemental formulas (100% free amino acids) are Neocate One+®, Neocate Junior®, and Vivonex Pediatric®. Splash E028® is also available as a flavor-free amino acid medical food supplement for children.

ENTERAL FORMULAS FOR CHILDREN OVER 10 YEARS OF AGE

Refer to the guidelines outlined in Chapter V for EN formula selection. Careful analysis of both adult and pediatric products may be necessary to meet the needs of teenage patients. Some adolescent patients may need a combination of both adult and pediatric formulas, and calcium and/or iron supplementation may be necessary to meet their higher requirements.

FORMULAS FOR CHILDREN WITH INBORN ERRORS OF METABOLISM

Children with inborn errors of metabolism require specialized EN formulas. For more information on these products, contact the Pediatric Metabolic registered dietitians (outpatient, phone 734-936-9213; inpatient, phone 734-764-9504).

MODULAR FORMULAS

A modular formula or a module is available in powder or liquid forms of individual macronutrients (protein, carbohydrate, fat) used to supplement the EN formula in order to meet a nutritional goal that is originally supplied by the original EN product. The mixing process of modulars may increase the risk for bacterial contamination and incorrect preparation. Further, the addition of modular supplements alters the caloric distribution in the formula and also results in a more concentrated formula with higher osmolality that may negatively impact feeding tolerance. Enteral modular supplements available on Formulary include protein (ProStat 64®; Prosource®), carbohydrates (Polycose®), and fat (Microlipid® [4.5 kcal/mL]; MCT oil [115 kcal/15 mL]) (Appendix M). Contact the registered dietitian on service for assistance with the choice of modular and for appropriate mixing and delivery of EN formulas.

ENTERAL NUTRITION REGIMEN

The preferred method of feeding children less than 1 year of age is by intermittent feeding to mimic nipple feeds and allow postprandial hormonal secretion. Intermittent feeding may be provided with a combination of nipple and gavage feeding to allow stimulation of oral motor skills while providing optimal nutrition. Continuous feeding may be better tolerated initially, especially in patients who have been on bowel rest for extended time, or in those who have a history of feeding intolerance. Continuous feeding should be used for all patients receiving EN into the small intestines.

Generally, the gastrointestinal tract tolerates increases in feeding volumes before it tolerate increases in formula osmolality. Most patients tolerate full-strength isotonic EN formulas at low administration rates. Current literature supports the use of a feeding protocol for preterm infants to promote consistency of practice and decrease the incidence of necrotizing enterocolitis. In the absence of a feeding protocol, the guidelines in Table 1 can be used to initiate EN in preterm infants. Certain practices and some literature support providing only "trophic feedings" (minimal feeding to test for gastrointestinal tolerance and to maintain intestinal functionality and integrity) in very low birthweight infants (weight less than 1500 g) for about 10 days or less without feeding advancement, to avoid the risk of feeding intolerance or necrotizing enterocolitis.

Table 1. Guidelines for Initiating Enteral Nutrition for Preterm Infants

Birth weight (g)	≤ 1000	> 1000– < 1250	1250– 1500	> 1500– 2000	> 2000– 2500
Volume of first feeding Schedule of feeding	10–20 mL/kg/day	10–20 mL/kg/day	20 mL/kg/day	20 mL/kg/day	5 mL every 3 hours
Volume rate of feeding advances	10–20 mL/kg/day	10–20 mL/kg/day	20 mL/kg/day	20 mL/kg/day may advance, as tolerated	5 mL every other feed as tolerated

For term infants, older children, and adolescents, the following approach is used for providing intermittent and continuous EN:

1. Determine the energy, protein, vitamin, mineral, and fluid requirements.
2. For term infants, determine the volume of human milk or formula to meet these requirements.
3. For intermittent feeding, initiate EN at a rate of 2 to 5 mL/kg every 3 to 4 hours. Advance the feeding rate in increments of 2 to 5 mL/kg every two

feedings to goal rate, as tolerated. Check for feeding residuals before each intermittent feeding. Hold EN if the residual volume is greater than twice the volume previously administered. Recheck for residuals in one hour, and restart intermittent feedings at the previous rate if residuals are decreased.

4. For continuous feeding, initiate EN at a rate of 1 to 2 mL/kg/hr. Advance continuous feeding to goal rate by 1 to 2 mL/kg every 8 to 12 hours, as tolerated. The initial feeding rate should not exceed 55 mL/hr, regardless of the child's age or body weight. Hold EN if the residual volume is greater than twice the hourly rate. Recheck for residuals in one hour, and restart continuous feeding at the previous rate if residuals are decreased.

5. For adolescents, EN can be started at a rate of 25 to 50 mL/hr, depending on anticipated gastrointestinal tolerance. Advance EN to goal rate in increments of 20 to 25 mL/hr every 8 to 12 hours, as tolerated.

6. Do not advance feeding rate and strength simultaneously.

HANG TIME FOR ENTERAL NUTRITION FORMULAS

To reduce microbial contamination, the hang time for reconstituted EN formulas is a maximum of 4 hours. The same hang time applies for human milk, and if a modular is added to the formula. Human milk should be hung for the shortest time possible. After one hour, the fat in human milk binds to the feeding tube, which would decrease the calorie intake to the infant. Therefore, it is best to administer human milk in small quantities by intermittent feeding boluses. If Human Milk Fortifier is added to human milk, the hang time of the final reconstituted formula is shortened to 2 hours. The maximum hang time for full-strength open-system EN formulas is 8 hours.

MONITORING PARAMETERS

Because frequent blood draws in children can lead to anemia of blood loss, measurement of biochemical nutritional markers (e.g., serum albumin, prealbumin, triglycerides, trace elements, and vitamin concentrations) should be coordinated with other laboratory draws to minimize blood loss. Serum electrolyte concentrations should be regularly assessed along with the monitoring of clinical status.

Other parameters that should be regularly monitored include intake and output, body weight, number and consistency of stools, signs of abdominal distention, feeding residuals, and the position of tube feeding. Tube feeding position is confirmed by a low upright chest X-ray. Check the penmark on the tube that denotes the exit point from the nares at the time of initial tube placement, or measure the length of the tube exiting from the nares. Check tube position every 4 hours for continuous feeding or prior to each intermittent feeding. Notify the physician if tube migration is suspected.

Interruptions in tube feeding administration should be documented and the reason specified (e.g., procedures, high residual volumes, clogged feeding tube).

COMPLICATIONS ASSOCIATED WITH ENTERAL FEEDING

Chapter XI provides details on the complications of EN and their management. If complications prevent adequate EN for more than 2 to 3 days in infants and children, and for about 5 to 7 days in well-nourished adolescents, then PN should be considered.

ORAL MEDICATION ADMINISTRATION DURING ENTERAL FEEDING

Whenever possible, medications should be administered orally to prevent the occlusion of the feeding tube. If a medication is to be administered through the feeding tube, an oral liquid medication should be used when available. Elixirs and oral suspensions should be diluted with water before administration. Each medication should be administered separately, flushing the feeding tube with 5 mL of water before and after each medication administration.

Oral medications that should not be crushed include sublingual, buccal, enteric-coated, and extended-release forms. Some medications should not be crushed because they can cause irritation to the oral mucosa, are extremely bitter, or stain the teeth. A list of oral medications that should not be crushed is shown in Appendix F.

X. PARENTERAL NUTRITION FOR PEDIATRIC PATIENTS

Three different parenteral nutrition (PN) order sets are used for pediatric patients based on body weight, and include: PN for less than 10 kg (neonatal), between 10 and 30 kg (pediatric), and greater than 30 kg (adolescents). PN components include macronutrients (amino acids, dextrose, intravenous lipid emulsions) fluids, electrolytes, and micronutrients (multivitamins, trace elements).

MACRONUTRIENTS

Amino Acids

Amino acids are used for body protein synthesis and lean body mass accretion. Amino acids are also a source of calories, providing 4 kcal/g. Amino acids usually contribute to about 10% to 15% of total daily calories in pediatric PN. Adequate calories from dextrose and intravenous lipid emulsions must be provided with proteins to optimize nitrogen retention. Protein requirements for pediatric patients are shown in Chapter VIII.

Parenteral amino acid solutions for low birthweight infants are formulated to produce plasma amino acid concentrations comparable to those of the postprandial breastfed infants of similar gestational age. Trophamine[®] 10% is the crystalline amino acid bulk solution available on Formulary for use in the PN of infants whose body weight is less than 10 kg. FreAmine III[®] 10% is the parenteral amino acid bulk solution Formulary product of choice for use in the PN of patients whose body weight exceeds 10 kg. Unlike FreAmine III[®] 10%, Aminosyn II[®] 15% contains no phosphate and is available for use in patients with persistent hyperphosphatemia despite restrictions in phosphate intake. The parenteral crystalline amino acid bulk solutions available on Formulary are shown in Appendix H.

Dextrose

Dextrose (d-glucose) is a source of calories and carbon skeletons for tissue growth. Hydrous dextrose has a caloric value of 3.4 kcal/g, and typically contributes about 50% to 60% of total daily calories in PN. Dextrose utilization rate in the pediatric population ranges from 4 to 14 mg/kg/min, depending on patient age, weight, tolerance, and metabolic state. Decreased dextrose utilization occurs during stress (e.g., sepsis, organ dysfunction; post-surgery) and with corticosteroid therapy. In neonates, dextrose infusion rate (DIR) is initiated at 4 to 8 mg/kg/min and advanced at a daily rate of 2 mg/kg/min until the nutritional goal is reached, with a maximum DIR of 14 mg/kg/min. A minimum DIR of 4 mg/kg/min is required in neonates to spare body proteins from being used for energy. CareLink automatically calculates the DIR in PN based on the following:

$$DIR \text{ (mg/kg/min)} = \frac{\text{Total dextrose (mg)}}{\text{Body weight (kg)} \times (1{,}440 \text{ min})^a}$$

[a]24 hours = 1,440 minutes

Exceeding the maximum DIR could result in hyperglycemia. Preterm infants are especially are at high risk for hyperglycemia because of decreased number and function of their insulin receptors and the immaturity of their metabolic pathways. Most term infants and children can tolerate dextrose concentrations in PN starting at 10% (100 g/L) and increasing daily by 2.5% to 5% until the goal dextrose calories are reached. The final dextrose concentration in pediatric peripheral PN admixtures is limited to 12.5% (125 g/L). Phlebitis and superficial skin slough are the most common complications in patients receiving peripheral PN. For central vein administration, dextrose concentration in PN can be increased up to 35% (350 g/L).

In low birthweight and critically ill infants, umbilical artery catheters (UAC) and umbilical vein catheters (UVC) are often used for PN infusion. Central PN admixtures with dextrose concentrations exceeding 12.5% can be infused through a UVC, once placement of the catheter tip above the diaphragm is confirmed. Dextrose concentrations should be limited to a maximum of 12.5% when infused through a UAC. A peripherally inserted central catheter (PICC) may be placed once the UAC and UVC are removed.

The infusion of PN admixtures should be tapered off slowly over 1 to 2 hours before it is stopped to avoid reactive hypoglycemia. If the PN is quickly discontinued, dextrose 10% or 12.5% in water solutions should be infused in place of PN.

Intravenous Lipid Emulsions

Intravenous lipid emulsions are a source of calories and essential fatty acids (linoleic acid, α-linolenic acid). The 20% intravenous lipid emulsion available on Formulary is Liposyn III 20%[®] and provides 2 kcal/mL. Intravenous lipid emulsions usually provide 20% to 30% of total daily calories in PN. The 20% lipid emulsion has better clearance than the 10% emulsion due to its lower phospholipid-to-triglyceride ratio (0.06 vs. 0.12, respectively). Chapter VI provides details on the composition and metabolism of intravenous lipid emulsions.

Intravenous lipid emulsion particles are mainly metabolized by the lipoprotein lipase enzyme in the bloodstream. The activity of the lipoprotein lipase enzyme is capacity-limited; its activity is decreased in critically ill patients, and its availability is limited in premature neonates possibly due to limited fat stores. Intravenous lipid emulsions in infants and children are usually initiated at 1 g/kg/day and advanced to a maximum of 3 g/kg/day. In case of hypertriglyceridemia, a lower average dose of intravenous lipid emulsions at 0.5 to 1 g/kg/day should be administered to prevent essential fatty acid deficiency. In infants and children with serum triglyceride concentrations that exceed 275 mg/dL, intermittent rather than daily infusion of intravenous lipid emulsions should be provided few times a week.

The safety of intravenous lipid emulsions in preterm infants with hyperbilirubinemia is controversial. There is a concern about the development of kernicterus as bilirubin may be displaced from its albumin binding sites by free fatty acids.

FLUIDS

Guidelines for maintenance fluid requirements for pediatric patients are listed in Tables 1 and 2. Fluid requirements are increased with higher insensible water losses (e.g., extremely low birthweight infants, phototherapy, gastroschisis, and omphalocele). Fluids should be administered cautiously during the first days of life of premature neonates with respiratory distress syndrome, because it may increase the risk of developing patent ductus arteriosus.

Table 1. Daily Fluid Recommendations in Newborn Infants

Day of life	Weight ≤ 1250 g	Weight > 1250 g	Term Infant
	Fluid volume (mL/kg/day)		
1	80	80	60–80
2	80–100	80–100	70–90
3	a	a	80–100
4	a	a	100–120
≥ 5	a	a	120–140

a = Increase fluid intake as needed to meet calorie requirements.

Table 2. Daily Maintenance Fluid Requirements for Children Older than One Month of Age

Body Weight (kg)	Fluid
1–10	100 mL/kg/day
10–20	1000 mL + 50 mL for each kg over 10 kg
> 20	1500 mL + 20 mL for each kg over 20 kg

ELECTROLYTES

Electrolytes are essential factors in biochemical and enzymatic reactions (e.g., cell membrane structure and function, growth, neurotransmission, muscle contraction, cardiovascular function, bone composition, hormone function, and fluid homeostasis). Electrolytes additions are added in salt forms to the PN and include sodium, potassium, phosphorus (as phosphate), calcium, magnesium, chloride, and acetate (Table 3). Electrolyte supplementation in PN admixtures is guided by serum electrolyte concentrations, considering renal function, gastrointestinal losses, fluid shifts, acid-base status, and medication therapy. Acute electrolyte losses should be replaced outside the PN admixture.

Calcium-Phosphate Solubility

Strict compatibility guidelines are followed to prevent calcium-phosphate precipitation in PN admixtures. Limited amounts of calcium and phosphorus can be provided in neonatal PN admixtures. CareLink (Computerized Prescriber Order Entry, CPOE) automatically calculates the calcium and phosphate limits in PN. Chapter VI provides details on the chemical and physical conditions that affect calcium and phosphate solubility in PN admixtures. The following guidelines are followed to determine the maximum amount of calcium and phosphorus that can be safely added into the neonatal PN admixture:

1. Calculate the percent of amino acids in the neonatal PN admixture:

$$\% \text{ Amino acids} = \frac{\text{g/kg amino acids x body weight (kg)}}{\text{PN volume (mL)}} \times 100$$

2. Determine from the chart, below, the maximum corresponding precipitation factor (PPT) in the PN admixture that can be used in relation to the calculated % AA:

% Amino acids	PPT
> 1.5%	≤ 3
1–1.5%	≤ 2
< 1%	Calcium or phosphate is only added

3. PPT (use the maximum factor allowed to maximize calcium and phosphate intake):

$$\text{PPT} = \frac{\text{calcium (mEq/kg) + phosphate (mmol/kg)}}{\text{PN volume (mL)}} \times \text{Weight (kg)} \times 100$$

4. A calcium-to-phosphate ratio of 2 to 2.6 mEq-to-1 mmol is desirable in PN to achieve optimal bone calcium and phosphate retention. This ratio can also be expressed as 1.3 to 1.7 mg of calcium-to-1 mg of phosphate. A ratio of 2-to-1 is recommended for low birthweight infants.

Chloride and Acetate

The chloride-to-acetate ratio can be adjusted to the patient's acid-base status. Acetate is converted in vivo to bicarbonate, likely outside the liver. Chloride is largely excreted by the kidneys. The standard chloride-to-acetate ratio is 1.5 to 1. In case of alkalemia, a high chloride-to-low-acetate ratio is used. In case of bicarbonate deficit, a low chloride-to-high-acetate ratio is used. Chloride and acetate adjustments in PN should be followed with close monitoring of the patient's acid-base status and serum potassium concentrations, especially in premature neonates who have poor response to acid-base changes because of their kidneys inefficiency to handle bicarbonate and hydrogen ions.

VITAMINS

Parenteral pediatric multivitamins are formulated based on the guidelines of the American Medical Association for vitamin supplements. Vitamins are cofactors in multiple metabolic reactions. Metabolic stress conditions increase metabolic demands and could result in vitamin depletion, especially water-soluble vitamins, if they are not adequately supplemented. Therefore, daily vitamin supplementation in PN admixtures is essential for proper metabolism, tissue healing, and to prevent vitamin deficiencies.

Thiamine deficiency, resulting in lactic acidosis and deaths, occurred in patients who received thiamine-free PN during periodic nationwide multivitamin shortages. Thiamine deficiency without adequate thiamine supplementation may occur very early with the dextrose load in PN that increases the needs for thiamine. Based on the Centers for Disease Control (CDC, MMWR Weekly June 13, 1997;46(23);523-8) report, the time for development of severe lactic acidosis in those reports ranged from 7 to 34 days, which is consistent with the required time to deplete body thiamine stores in healthy adults deprived of this vitamin. The risk of thiamine deficiency could be higher following the initiation of nutrition support therapy in malnourished individuals with depleted thiamine stores. Thiamine is a water-soluble vitamin with limited body reserves, and is essential for the oxidation of pyruvate via the citric acid cycle. In case of thiamine deficiency, pyruvate is converted instead to lactate by the lactate dehydrogenase enzyme, which may cause lactate accumulation and lactic acidosis. Appendix A provides information on vitamin deficiency and toxicity, and laboratory parameters to monitor vitamin status.

Pediatric intravenous multivitamin formulations (Infuvite Pediatric®) contain a combination of fat- and water-soluble vitamins and are automatically added daily to the PN admixture (Table 4). Patients who weigh more than 30 kg receive the adult intravenous multivitamin formulation (Infuvite® Adult) (Chapter VI).

TRACE ELEMENTS

Daily supplementation of trace elements (zinc, copper, manganese, chromium, selenium) in PN admixtures ensures adequate substrate metabolism and contributes to the body repair process and normal resistance. Parenteral trace element formulations and supplementation are based on the 1988 recommendations for daily intravenous supplements of trace elements in the absence of deficiencies by the Nutrition Advisory Group of the American Medical Association and the Society of Clinical Nutrition. The pediatric formulation of the multiple trace element injection (Multitrace[®]-4-Pediatric) available on Formulary is shown in Table 5. Multitrace[®] 4-Pediatric 0.2 mL/kg/day with additional selenium 3 mcg/kg/day is automatically added to the daily PN of pediatric patients, unless otherwise indicated. These recommendations were questioned by the Safe Practice Guidelines by the American Society for Parenteral and Enteral Nutrition (A.S.P.E.N.) that published different guidelines for daily parenteral trace element supplementation in pediatric PN admixtures (Table 6).

Table 3. Daily Electrolytes Maintenance Requirements and Concentration Limits in Parenteral Nutrition for Pediatric Patients

Electrolyte	Daily requirements	Maximum electrolyte concentration in PN admixture (per 1000 mL)
Body weight < 10 kg		
Sodium	2–8 mEq/kg	154 mEq
Potassium	2–4 mEq/kg	120 mEq
Chloride	2–5 mEq/kg	Wide range[a]
Acetate	Variable[a]	Wide range[a]
Calcium	1–3 mEq/kg	Variable[b]
Phosphorus	0.5–2 mmol/kg	Variable[b]
Magnesium	0.25–1 mEq/kg	20 mEq
Body weight 10–30 kg		
Sodium	20–150 mEq	154 mEq
Potassium	20–120 mEq	120 mEq
Chloride	20–150 mEq	Wide range[a]
Acetate	20–120 mEq	Wide range[a]
Calcium	5–20 mEq	Variable[b]
Phosphorus	4–24 mmol	Variable[b]
Magnesium	4–24 mEq	20 mEq

[a]Chloride-to-acetate ratio adjusted based on the patient's acid-base status.
[b]Dependent on calcium and phosphorus solution content.

Table 4. Composition and Dosing of Pediatric Intravenous Multivitamin

Vitamin	Infuvite Pediatric[®]
Fat-soluble vitamins	
Vitamin A	2300 IU
Vitamin D	400 IU
Vitamin E	7 IU
Vitamin K	200 mcg
Water-soluble vitamins	
Thiamine (B1)	1.2 mg
Riboflavin (B2)	1.4 mg
Niacin (B3)	17 mg
Pantothenic acid (B5)	5 mg
Pyridoxine (B6)	1 mg
Cyanocobalamin (B12)	1 mcg
Biotin (H)	20 mcg
Folate	140 mcg
Ascorbic acid (C)	80 mg
Dose	Weight: $\geq$ 1750 g, 5 mL/day; < 1750 g, 3.3 mL/day

Table 5. Composition and Dosing of PTE-4[®] for Pediatrics Patients[a]

Multitrace[®] 4-Pediatric	Zinc (sulfate)	Copper (sulfate)	Manganese (sulfate)	Chromium (chloride)
1 mL	1 mg	0.1 mg	25 mcg	1 mcg
0.2 mL	0.2 mg	0.02 mg	5 mcg	0.2 mcg
Dose: 0.2 mL/kg/day[b]				

[a]Selenium (as selenious acid) 3 mcg/kg/day is added with the Multitrace[®] 4-Pediatric to PN.
[b]Unless otherwise indicated.

Chapter VI describes the multiple trace elements injection formulation (Multitrace[®] 5-Concentrate) used in the PN for adolescents, the single trace element formulations available on Formulary, and the metabolic functions of trace elements. Chapter XII provides details on metabolic complications of trace elements in patients receiving PN.

Table 6. Daily Parenteral Trace Element Requirements in Parenteral Nutrition for Children and Neonates, According to A.S.P.E.N. Guidelines

Age group	Zinc	Copper	Manganese	Chromium	Selenium
Preterm infant (mcg/kg/day)	400	20	1	0.05–0.3	1.5–4.5
Term infant 3–10 kg (mcg/kg/day)	50–250	20	1	0.2	2
Children 10–40 kg (mcg/kg/day)	50–125	5–20	1	0.14–0.2	1–2
Maximum daily dose	5 mg	300 mcg	50 mcg	5 mcg	30 mcg

MEDICATION ADDITIVES TO PARENTERAL NUTRITION ADMIXTURES

Histamine-2 Receptor Antagonists

Histamine-2 receptor antagonists (H_2RAs) are compatible with PN admixtures. Concerns exist about the possible association between ranitidine and the occurrence of necrotizing enterocolitis in very low birthweight infants (weight less than 1500 g). Neonates weighing less than 1250 g will receive H_2RAs only if the benefits of H_2RAs outweigh the risks. The entire 24-hour dose can be added to the daily PN admixture (Table 7).

Table 7. Usual Dose of Continuous Intravenous H_2RA Infusion in Infants and Children

Intravenous H_2RA dose[a]	Infants < 2–3 weeks of age	Children
Ranitidine[b]	1–2 mg/kg/day	2–4 mg/kg/day
Famotidine	0.5 mg/kg/day	0.5 mg/kg/day

[a]Doses vary with clinical condition. Dose reduction is indicated with renal impairment.
[b]Maximum ranitidine dose is 6 mg/kg/day per PN bag for pediatric patients.

Heparin

Heparin is no longer routinely added to PN admixtures, mainly because of the risk for heparin-induced thrombocytopenia. Heparin is a cofactor of the lipoprotein lipase enzyme that enhances the clearance of intravenous lipid emulsions in the bloodstream (post-heparin lipolytic activity). A low dose heparin added to the PN admixture may prevent platelet thrombin and clots formation at the intravenous catheter tip, although the supporting evidence remains inconclusive. Exceptions when heparin 0.5 unit/mL may be added to the PN admixture is in the neonatal intensive care unit, to maintain intravenous catheter patency if the neonate has a peripherally inserted central catheter (PICC) with a PN infusion rate less than 10 mL/hr, or a tunneled catheter with PN infusion rate less than 3 mL/hr.

Regular Human Insulin

Insulin therapy is difficult to regulate in infants, and the risk of serum glucose concentrations exceeding 200 mg/dL is uncommon. Preterm infants may have variability in glucose autoregulation, which places them at risk for hyperglycemia or hypoglycemia. Therefore, insulin therapy for a safe and adequate glucose control can best be achieved via continuous insulin infusion (or subcutaneous insulin when indicated), rather than adding insulin to PN.

In older children and adolescents, regular human insulin may be added to the PN admixture. Once serum glucose concentrations stabilize, 70% of the average sliding scale insulin or continuous insulin infusion requirements can be added to the PN admixture. The insulin dose is adjusted afterwards as needed, based on serum glucose concentrations. To avoid hypoglycemia, adjustments to the insulin dose should be made as dictated by scheduled monitoring of capillary or serum glucose concentrations, especially when the metabolic stress level is decreasing, pancreatitis is resolving, and when corticosteroid doses are tapered or discontinued.

Parenteral Iron

Iron is not a component of PN. Iron deficiency may occur in patients with malabsorption disorders and growing children who are chronically dependent on PN. Only sodium chloride-containing iron products should be used intravenously. Phenol-containing iron products are for intramuscular use only. Iron dextran is the only parenteral iron product that can be added to the lipid-free PN admixture. Iron dextran should only be used when the oral route is not feasible, intestinal iron absorption is unreliable, or with gastrointestinal intolerance to oral iron supplements. Iron replacement therapy is not an emergency. Parenteral iron should be avoided in infected patients due to concerns of increased bacterial proliferation because bacteria may use iron for growth.

Immediate or delayed anaphylaxis with severe hypersensitivity reactions (characterized by cardiovascular collapse, cardiac arrest, bronchospasm, dyspnea, angioedema, urticaria, muscle spasm), fevers, chills, backache, myalgia, dizziness, syncope, and rash have been reported with iron dextran therapy. Prior to addition to the PN admixture, an intravenous test dose of iron dextran mixed in 0.9% sodium chloride should be administered over 15 to 30 minutes to determine susceptibility to adverse reactions. One hour should elapse before administering the remaining initial dose.

Although parenteral iron manufacturers do not recommend iron dextran to be given in the first 4 months of life, studies have reported its safety and efficacy in neonates. Daily doses of iron dextran up to 1 mg/kg have been added to neonatal PN admixtures to prevent iron deficiency anemia. The total replacement dose of iron dextran in children for iron deficiency anemia not due to blood loss is calculated as follows:

Iron dextran (mL) = 0.0476 x body weight (kg) x [desired hemoglobin (g/dL) – observed hemoglobin (g/dL)] + 1 mL per 5 kg of body weight (up to a maximum of14 mL)

1 mL of iron dextran = 50 mg of elemental iron

Desired hemoglobin (g/dL) = 12, if patient weighs less than 15 kg; or 14.8 if patient weighs more than 15 kg

The total dose of iron dextran is divided in equal increments and administered with the maximum daily dose based on the patient's body weight:

Infants weight, less than 5 kg: 25 mg (0.5 mL) iron dextran

Children weight, 5 to 10 kg: 50 mg (1 mL) iron dextran

Children weight, more than 10 kg: 100 mg (2 mL) iron dextran

The daily dose up to 100 mg of iron dextran may be added to each 24-hour supply of non-lipid containing PN admixture, until the total iron replacement dose is administered. Iron dextran is incompatible in-solution and at the Y-injection site with intravenous lipid emulsions causing the emulsion to "oil out."

Other parenteral iron formulations, including iron sucrose and sodium ferric gluconate, have not been evaluated for compatibility with PN admixtures and should not be added or co-infused with PN admixtures. Iron sucrose and sodium ferric gluconate are associated with lower rate of serious hypersensitivity reactions compared to iron dextran and do not usually require a test dose.

Iron and Epoetin Use in Anemia of Prematurity

Iron supplementation (oral or parenteral) is essential for the optimal effects of epoetin alpha (EPO) unless iron stores are already in excess. Although it is not an approved indication, EPO has been used in very low birthweight infants as an alternative to transfusion therapy for the treatment of anemia of prematurity. EPO can be given intravenously or subcutaneously, and variable dosing regimens have been used including: 25 to 100 units/kg/dose administered 3 times per week; 100 units/kg/dose 5 times per week; or 200 units/kg/dose every other day for a total of 10 doses. Serum iron concentrations, ferritin, and total iron binding capacity should be evaluated before EPO therapy. Blood pressure, renal function, hematocrit, transferrin saturation, serum iron concentrations and ferritin should be monitored during EPO therapy.

CARNITINE

Carnitine is a quaternary amine required for the transport of long-chain fatty acids into the mitochondria where they undergo oxidation to generate energy. Carnitine is not a standard component of PN. Although carnitine is endogenously synthesized from methionine and lysine in the liver and kidneys, preterm infants are at risk for carnitine deficiency due to their limited tissue carnitine reserves and reduced capacity for carnitine biosynthesis. Low plasma carnitine concentrations have been associated with reduced fatty acid oxidation, possibly leading to hypertriglyceridemia. However, even with normal plasma carnitine concentrations hypertriglyceridemia can still occur, thereby questioning the exact role of carnitine on serum triglyceride concentrations.

Oral L-carnitine is well absorbed and achieves similar plasma carnitine concentrations to intravenous L-carnitine. Supplementation of L-carnitine in PN and EN improves fatty acid oxidation, nitrogen balance, and weight gain in infants. Although the optimal dose and duration of L-carnitine to achieve these effects are not well defined, clinical studies in neonates and infants have shown that L-carnitine doses at 10 to 20 mg/kg/day are sufficient to normalize plasma carnitine concentrations. The administration of L-carnitine at 20 mg/kg/day for 8 weeks to neonates resulted in plasma total carnitine concentrations that exceeded the normal plasma carnitine reference range. Therefore, L-carnitine doses exceeding 20 mg/kg/day in infants may unlikely be of clinical benefit. Although L-carnitine supplementation is generally safe, large oral L-carnitine doses have caused seizures in patients who may or may not have had underlying seizure disorders, in addition to diarrhea, nausea, and abdominal cramps. Further, there are concerns that high L-carnitine doses may have a negative effect on neonatal growth, possibly by increasing the infant's metabolic rate. L-carnitine doses of 48 mg/kg/day in PN of low birthweight infants increased protein oxidation, decreased nitrogen balance, and increased the time to regain birth weight. L-carnitine 5 mg/kg/day are routinely added to the PN of neonates who weigh less than 1500 g in the neonatal intensive care unit. L-carnitine doses in pediatric patients with acquired secondary carnitine deficiency should not exceed 20 mg/kg/day. Higher L-carnitine doses may be required in patients treated with haemodialysis or continuous renal replacement therapy (CRRT) because of carnitine losses across the hemodiafilter.

The optimal duration of parenteral L-carnitine supplementation for patients with acquired secondary carnitine deficiency is unknown, but can be guided by periodic monitoring of plasma carnitine concentrations. Monitoring plasma total and free carnitine and acylcarnitine (intermediate in fatty acid oxidation) concentrations is recommended whenever L-carnitine is supplemented in PN admixtures or whenever carnitine deficiency is suspected. Serum triglyceride concentrations should be measured when L-carnitine is used to correct hypertriglyceridemia.

STARTER PARENTERAL NUTRITION FOR VERY LOW BIRTHWEIGHT NEONATES

The very low birthweight infant (birthweight less than 1500 g) is born with limited nutritional reserves and could become rapidly malnourished after being deprived for some time after birth from the nutrients supplied while a fetus. Very low birthweight infants also have continuous protein loss in desquamated epidermal cells and urine (as urea), are significantly more catabolic than term infants, can quickly use their body proteins for energy, and experience a decrease in amino acid levels following birth.

Early adequate nutrition of the very low birthweight infant is crucial, and aims at providing uninterrupted nutrients to the infant in the transition from fetal to extrauterine life, in order to prevent somatic growth failure and neurodevelopment delays. Early (within 24 hours after birth) intake of parenteral amino acids at doses up to 3.8 to 4 g/kg/day in very low birthweight infants improves protein balance and nitrogen retention, and may stimulate insulin release to avoid hyperglycemia that is believed to be partially caused by irrepressible increased endogenous glucose production.

Protein and calories are essential for growth, but must be provided in appropriate proportions for their optimal utilization. The majority of very low birthweight infants receive PN because of their immature gastrointestinal tract that precludes enteral feeding. Therefore, prompt initiation of PN within a few hours after birth is essential. The "starter PN" is available to use in very low birthweight infants in the neonatal intensive care unit who weigh 1500 g or less, for whom obtaining PN during the off hours of the compounding Pharmacy is not possible. The next day, PN follows the procedures of regular PN ordering. The "starter PN" formulation for low birthweight neonates is as follows:

Starter PN for very low birthweight infants

Total volume	100 mL
Amino acids (Trophamine® 10%)	3% (3 g)
Dextrose	10% (10 g)
Multivitamins (M.V.I. Pediatric®)	3.3 mL
Inherent electrolytes (per 100 mL)	Sodium 0.15 mEq
	Chloride < 0.1 mEq
	Acetate 2.91 mEq)
Osmolarity	~ 800 mOsm/L

Two "starter PN" bags are stocked at any given time in Mott Children's Pharmacy under refrigeration, with an expiration time of 14 days. Intravenous multivitamins are added to the "starter PN" admixture before dispensing. Intravenous lipid emulsions can also be dispensed by the Pharmacy with the "starter PN" when requested.

STARTER PARENTERAL NUTRITION FOR PATIENTS WITH UREA CYCLE DISORDERS

Urea cycle disorders are inborn errors of metabolism caused by enzymatic deficiency in the urea cycle pathway that transforms nitrogen to urea. Urea cycle disorders are associated with increased blood ammonia levels, which may present with a variety of neurologic (e.g., altered mental status, decreased consciousness, seizures, abnormal motor function) and gastrointestinal (e.g., vomiting, nausea, diarrhea, poor feeding tolerance, constipation) symptoms. During their acute presentation, patients are typically catabolic and oral feedings are not always possible. Therefore, early PN is indicated with minimal protein intake to avoid worsening of hyperammonemia while reducing the impact of catabolism on skeletal protein losses.

When indicated, a "starter PN" formulation can be made available on-demand to patients with urea cycle disorders for whom obtaining PN during regular hours of the compounding Pharmacy is not possible. Ordering the "starter PN" for patients with urea cycle disorders is restricted to physicians (or designate) from the Genetics Service. These orders can be found in CareLink under the Genetics Order Set for urea cycle defects. The "starter PN" formulation for patients with inborn errors of metabolism is shown in Table 8.

Table 8. Starter Parenteral Nutrition Formulation for Patients with Urea Cycle Disorders

Patient weight	Amino acid dose[a]	Dextrose concentration[b]	Sodium chloride	Parenteral MVI
< 10 kg	0.5–1 g/kg/day	12.5%	q.s. to 40 mEq/L	5 mL/day[c]
10–30 kg	0.5–1 mg/kg/day	10%	q.s. to 150 mEq/L	5 mL/day[c]
> 30 kg	0.5–1 mg/kg/day	10%	q.s. to 150 mEq/L	10 mL/day[d]

MVI = multivitamins.
[a]Trophamine® 10% is used for all patient weight categories. This bulk solution contains inherent
electrolytes including sodium 5 mEq/L, acetate 97 mEq/L, and chloride < 3 mEq/L.
[b]Dextrose concentration 12.5% = 12.5 g/100 mL; 10% = 10 g/100 mL.
[c]Pediatric intravenous multivitamin (M.V.I. Pediatric®).
[d]Adult intravenous multivitamin (Infuvite® Adult).

The "starter PN" formulation is compounded in Mott Pharmacy (phone 734-764-8208) and will be available to the patient within 4 hours after order initiation. The "starter PN" admixture should be administered at the prescribed infusion rate, should be discarded after 24 hours, and cannot be re-ordered for a second time for the same patient. The next day, obtaining PN follows the procedures of regular PN ordering.

TRANSITION FROM PARENTERAL TO ENTERAL NUTRITION OR ORAL DIET

The transition from PN to EN should be gradual and closely monitored to ensure that patients continue to adequately receive their nutritional requirements.

The preferred method of reintroducing EN is via continuous enteral feeding over 24 hours. Once a patient tolerates 50% of the desired hourly volume, the PN infusion rate is decreased proportionally by 50%. PN is discontinued once the patient is tolerating 75% of the desired hourly rate of EN.

For patients transitioning to oral diet, calorie counts can be ordered to quantify the oral calorie and protein intake. Calorie counts begin the next day and continue for 2 or 3 days. Calories in PN are adjusted according to the calorie count results, and PN is tapered off accordingly. PN is discontinued once a patient tolerates 75% of the desired oral calorie and protein requirements.

XI. COMPLICATIONS ASSOCIATED WITH ENTERAL NUTRITION

A number of complications can occur with enteral nutrition (EN) or tube feeding that can be classified as gastrointestinal, metabolic, and mechanical (Table 1). Electrolyte imbalances are not discussed herein, and they primarily occur in the setting of diseases and with specific medication therapies (see Chapter XII).

Table 1. Complications Associated with Enteral Nutrition and Treatment

Complication	Possible causes	Suggested treatment
Gastrointestinal		
Diarrhea (6 to 8 loose watery stools daily)	Osmotic overload	Review oral medications for hypertonic elixirs, sorbitol-containing oral liquid medications, and antacids Dilute oral elixirs, and change to non-sorbitol containing oral liquid medications Provide continuous rather than bolus feeding Avoid overuse of anti-diarrheal medications
	Lactose intolerance	Monitor lactose intake if also taking oral diet
	Contaminated formula	Change EN bag and tubing every 24 hours Limit hang times to 4 hours for reconstituted or diluted EN formulas, and 8 hours for full-strength liquid EN formulas
	Nervous tension	Promote restful environment
	Oral medications	Review oral medications especially for antibiotics, antacids, and H_2 receptor antagonists as possible causes
	Intestinal infection	Rule out and treat *Clostridium difficile* infection Rule out and treat bacterial overgrowth if suspected
	Low residue feeding	Try using a fiber-enriched EN formula[a]
Nausea	Volume overload	Decrease feeding volume and/or flow rate
Vomiting	Obstruction, delayed gastric emptying, medication-induced	Rule out gastrointestinal obstruction Review medication therapies as possible causes

Complication	Possible causes	Suggested treatment
Cramping	Rapid feeding	Decrease feeding volume and/or flow rate Advance flow rate gradually over 48 to 72 hours or less
Delayed gastric emptying	Diabetes, gastric surgery, trauma, thermal injury, sepsis	Check GRV every 4 hours and return up to 200 mL into stomach If GRV is above 200 mL[b] on two successive checks, hold EN for 1 hour and recheck Consider duodenal or jejunal feedings
Constipation	Insufficient fluid intake	Increase fluid/water intake Try a fiber-enriched EN formula[a]
	Low residue feeding	Increase physical activity, as tolerated
	Decreased intestinal motility	Rule out intestinal obstruction, medication-induced dysmotility (e.g., opioids, dopamine), and metabolic causes (e.g., hypokalemia, hypomagnesemia) Treat constipation
	Excessive free water	Reduce free water (hypotonic, low-sodium fluids) intake
Dehydration	Insufficient free water	Increase fluid/water intake Administer additional free water daily based on fluid requirements and tolerance Monitor fluid intake and losses
	Diarrhea Vomiting	Refer to gastrointestinal complications
	Hyperglycemia	Monitor serum glucose concentrations, especially in diabetics, elderly, pancreatic disease, and treat with insulin if needed Rule out sepsis and medication therapies (e.g., corticosteroids) as possible causes
Overhydration	Excess fluid intake Acute kidney injury Chronic kidney disease	Decrease fluid volume intake, monitor losses Reassess appropriateness of EN formula Change to a calorie-dense EN formula
Refeeding syndrome	Severe malnutrition, significant weight loss	Prevention is key (see Chapter XII) Replace electrolytes aggressively Initiate EN at 25% of nutritional goal and advance over 3 to 5 days to goal rate
Mechanical Dislodged tube	Confused patient	Restrain patient, bridle tube, or place permanent feeding tube

Table 1 (continued). Complications Associated with Enteral Nutrition and Treatment

Complication	Possible causes	Suggested treatment
Obstructed tube[c]	Inadequate flushing	Flush tubes with 5 to 30 mL of water every 4 hours, before and after: medication administration, checking GRV, and stopping feeding[d]
	Medication in tablet dosage forms	Crush medications well or use liquid forms Administer medications orally, if possible Treatment: instill in tube a mixture of one capsule of pancrelipase with one crushed tablet of sodium bicarbonate dissolved in 5 mL of warm water. Clamp tube for 5 to 10 minutes then flush tube[c]
Aspiration	Rapid feeding	Decrease feeding rate Check GRV every 4 hours If GRV exceed 200 mL[b] on two successive checks, hold EN for 1 hour and recheck GRV
	Incorrect patient position	Raise head of bed to 30 to 45 degrees during continuous feeding and 1 hour after and during bolus feedings, unless a medical contraindication exists
	Feeding tube malposition	Confirm tube placement with low upright chest X-ray Feeding tube can come into the pharynx with coughing or other activity. If in doubt, check by aspiration, insuflation, or X-ray

GRV = gastric residual volume(s).

[a]Based on the American Society for Parenteral and Enteral Nutrition (A.S.P.E.N.) and Society for Critical Care Medicine (SCCM) 2009 Critical Care Guidelines, soluble and insoluble fibers should be avoided in patients with severe intestinal dysmotility or bowel ischemia. Insoluble fibers should be avoided in all critically ill patients. Examples of soluble fiber supplements include psyllium, calcium polycarbophil, methylcellulose, guar gum, and pectin. Examples of insoluble fibers include wheat and bran.

[b]Based on the American Society for Parenteral and Enteral Nutrition (A.S.P.E.N.) and Society for Critical Care Medicine (SCCM) 2009 Critical Care Guidelines, holding EN for GRV less than 500 mL, in the absence of other signs of intolerance, should be avoided.

[c]Factors known to contribute to clogging of feeding tube include: calorie-dense EN formulas; fiber-containing EN formulas; incompatible or improper medication administration via tube; small tube diameters; inadequate tube flushes; interactions between gastric acid and proteins in EN formula; and silicone-made compared to polyurethane-made tubes.

[d]Water is the best choice for a feeding tube flush solution. Carbonated beverages or cranberry juice should not be used and are not superior to water as tube flush solutions. Some practice recommendations are to use "purified water" (sterile, solute-free, non-pyrogenic water) for feeding tube flushes in critically ill, immunocompromised, and pediatric patients, especially when the safety of tap water (municipal or locally available water that meets drinking water regulations) cannot be ascertained.

XII. METABOLIC COMPLICATIONS ASSOCIATED WITH PARENTERAL NUTRITION

Parenteral Nutrition (PN) therapy can be associated with several metabolic complications that mostly relate to the patient's underlying disease(s) and clinical condition(s) or to the inappropriate PN formulation or regimen. These complications can be avoided or minimized by the judicious use of PN and by close laboratory and patient monitoring during the course of PN therapy. Appropriate monitoring and adjustment of PN therapy are essential to avoid complications. Relevant laboratory and clinical information should be reviewed every time a new PN prescription is to be written.

HYPERGLYCEMIA

Normal serum glucose concentrations are between 80 and 110 mg/dL. Mild transient elevation of serum glucose concentrations may occur during the first few days of PN initiation, but may not require treatment if random serum glucose concentrations do not exceed 150 mg/dL. Endogenous insulin secretion adjusts itself, and serum glucose concentrations usually return to normal as the dextrose infusion rate (DIR) is advanced to nutritional goal over the next 48 to 72 hours. Hyperglycemia in patients receiving PN can be caused by excessive dextrose infusion, patient underlying factors (e.g., stress, diabetes, pancreatic disease, sepsis), or medication therapies (e.g., corticosteroids, tacrolimus, octreotide, catecholamine vasopressors like dopamine and norepinephrine, theophylline in infants). Unexplained and sudden glucose intolerance may be the first sign of sepsis that may not be yet apparent.

Excessive dextrose infusion can result in hypertriglyceridemia, hepatic steatosis, and respiratory decompensation. Uncontrolled hyperglycemia can cause fluid and electrolyte disturbances, hyperglycemic hyperosmolar nonketotic syndrome, increased susceptibility to infection, and increased patient morbidity and mortality. In critically ill patients, serum glucose concentrations should be typically maintained between 110 and 150 mg/dL.

PN therapy should not be a cause of hyperglycemia when appropriate amounts of dextrose are infused. All sources of dextrose (e.g., intravenous medication diluents, dextrose-contain dialysate or replacement fluids) and carbohydrate intake (e.g., oral, enteral nutrition) should be considered when calculating the amounts of dextrose given to the patient. The maximum 24-hour DIR is 4 mg/kg/min in adult patients, and 14 mg/kg/min in infants. In very low birthweight infants, a DIR up to 20 mg/kg/min may be required, at times, to treat neonatal hypoglycemia or to promote adequate weight gain. Caution should be exercised when a DIR exceeds 14 mg/kg/min in infants, as hyperglycemia and fatty liver can occur with excessive dextrose intake.

In adult and adolescent patients, regular human insulin at a minimum dose of 10 units can be added to the PN bag, as some insulin adsorbs to the container and intravenous tubing. Insulin is adjusted as needed to control hyperglycemia with a maximum dose of 100 units/L of PN admixture. If a patient requires insulin more than 100 units/L of PN admixture, an insulin drip should then be initiated.

Preterm infants have variability in glucose regulation and are at increased risk for hyperglycemia that is caused possibly by the immaturity of hepatic and pancreatic response. Reducing the DIR in infants could result in compromising nutritional intake. If necessary, the DIR in infants can be decreased but not below 4 mg/kg/min, a rate necessary to spare body proteins in infants. For safety and efficacy reasons, insulin should not be added to the PN of infants. Rather, a continuous regular insulin infusion should be used with a typical insulin dose is 0.01 to 0.1 unit/kg/hr for hyperglycemic infants. Neonates, especially low birthweight infants, are very sensitive to insulin and should be started at the low end of infusion rate. Serum glucose and potassium concentrations should be closely monitored during insulin administration.

HYPOGLYCEMIA

Hypoglycemia in patients receiving PN may occur following the rapid reduction of PN infusion rate (reactive hypoglycemia) or as a result of excessive insulin dosing in PN (iatrogenic hypoglycemia). Symptoms of diaphoresis, confusion, or agitation in a patient receiving PN should alert the clinician to the possibility of hypoglycemia. In adults, hypoglycemia is managed initially with a bolus administration of dextrose 50% in water, followed if necessary by continuous infusion dextrose 10% in water. Serum glucose concentrations and clinical response dictate further management. When the PN admixture is to be discontinued or has run out, administration of dextrose 10% in water in adult patients should prevent symptomatic hypoglycemia. Slow tapering of the PN admixture (e.g., over 2 hours) may prevent reactive hypoglycemia that may occur as a result of sudden interruption of dextrose infusion while endogenous insulin secretion continues. Patients with diabetes, renal or liver impairment, hypothyroidism, or those with history of hypoglycemia, may be more at risk for reactive hypoglycemia. In adult patients, a single episode of severe hypoglycemia (serum glucose concentrations below 40 mg/dL) may be an independent risk factor for increased patient mortality.

Neonates and especially preterm infants are at increased risk for hypoglycemia due to the immaturity of their protective metabolic mechanisms. Neonatal hypoglycemia could result from decreased gluconeogenesis, glycogenolysis, and ketogenesis; limited glycogen stores; increased glucose utilization (e.g., sepsis, hyperthermia, growth hormone deficiency); or hyperinsulinemia. Prolonged and recurrent hypoglycemia may result in acute systemic and neurologic effects. In infants, hypoglycemia is managed with an initial intravenous bolus of dextrose 200 to 250 mg/kg (2 to 2.5 mL/kg of dextrose 10% in water given over 2 to 5 minutes), followed by continuous dextrose infusion (e.g., dextrose 10% or 12.5% in water) at 5 to 8 mg/kg/min. Antihypoglycemic agents may also be used, as indicated.

In older children, an initial intravenous bolus of dextrose 10% in water at a dose of 500 mg/kg is used to treat hypoglycemia, followed when clinically indicated by a continuous infusion of dextrose 10% or 12.5% in water.

HYPERTRIGLYCERIDEMIA

Triglycerides in the bloodstream do not circulate freely, but rather are transported in the forms of lipoproteins (e.g., chylomicrons, VLDL). Increased serum triglyceride concentrations in patients receiving PN is usually caused by excess dextrose infusion, administration of large amounts of intravenous lipid emulsions, or a defective clearance of lipid emulsions or fat metabolism. The National Cholesterol Education Program Adult Treatment Panel III (NCEP-ATP III) defines serum triglyceride concentrations less than 150 mg/dL as normal, 150 to 199 mg/dL as borderline high, 200 to 499 mg/dL as high, and over 500 mg/dL as very high. In practice, intravenous lipid emulsion infusion is held when serum triglyceride concentrations exceed 400 mg/dL in adult patients, and 275 mg/dL in pediatric patients.

Excess dextrose infusion or high carbohydrate loads can cause hypertriglyceridemia. Excess glucose is converted in the liver and skeletal muscles by the fatty acid synthetase and acetyl Co-A synthetase to fatty acids. Fatty acids bind to glycerol to form triglycerides. In case of hypertriglyceridemia with or without hyperglycemia and without overfeeding from intravenous lipid emulsions, a reduction in carbohydrate calories should be attempted first, to correct the hypertriglyceridemia. Serum triglyceride concentrations are re-checked in 48 hours. If hypertriglyceridemia persists, the intravenous lipid emulsion dose should then be decreased in half and the dextrose concentration should be increased to avoid inadequate nutrition delivery. The 20% intravenous lipid emulsion provides the advantage of being better cleared than the 10% lipid emulsion due to its lower phospholipid-to-triglyceride ratio (0.06 vs. 0.12, respectively). Extending the lipid infusion time and keeping the lipid infusion rate below 0.12 g/kg/hr improves lipid clearance and may reduce serum triglyceride concentrations.

Serum triglyceride concentrations are routinely measured about once weekly in patients receiving PN. Because intravenous lipid emulsions have a relatively short plasma half-life (about 30 minutes), about 80% of intravenous lipids are cleared within 60 minutes. Therefore, measuring serum triglyceride concentrations during intravenous lipid emulsion infusion (rather than interrupting the infusion and waiting for a few hours before blood sampling) provides valid information on serum triglyceride concentrations. Serum triglyceride concentrations should be closely and more frequently (e.g., every 1 or 2 days) monitored in patients treated with propofol for continuous sedation. Propofol is delivered in a 10% lipid emulsion. Lipid calories from propofol (1.1 kcal/mL) should be counted when designing a nutrition support therapy, and intravenous lipid emulsion infusion should be held when propofol is infusing. Patients with diabetes, sepsis, acute kidney injury, morbid obesity, and acute pancreatitis are at increased risk for hypertriglyceridemia. Patients with acute pancreatitis can receive lipid emulsions in the absence of hypertriglyceridemia. Medications that are also known to alter fat metabolism (e.g., sirolimus, cyclosporine, tacrolimus, corticosteroids) may also cause hypertriglyceridemia.

In neonates, lipid clearance is reduced with prematurity. Intravenous lipid emulsions in infants are initiated at a dose of 0.5 to 1 g/kg/day, and advanced at a rate of 0.5 to 1 g/kg/day to a maximum of 3 g/kg/day. Smaller doses could be used in preterm infants or those with sepsis due to reduced lipid clearance. If serum triglyceride concentrations exceed 200 mg/dL, the lipid emulsion dose should be decreased to 0.5 to 1 g/kg/day. A trial of carnitine supplementation at doses of 10 to 20 mg/kg/day may be attempted to improve lipid clearance in infants with persistent or unexplained hypertriglyceridemia.

ESSENTIAL FATTY ACID DEFICIENCY

Essential fatty acids are linoleic acid (C18:2ω-6) and α-linolenic acid (C18:3ω-3). Arachidonic acid (C20:4ω-6) is synthesized from linoleic acid, which makes it an essential fatty acid in case of linoleic acid deficiency. In adults, biochemical evidence of essential fatty acid deficiency may be seen with 1 to 2 weeks of lipid-free PN. Clinical signs and symptoms may appear as early as 3 to 4 weeks of lipid deprivation. Biochemical evidence of essential fatty acid deficiency, which usually precedes the appearance of clinical signs and symptoms, reveals low plasma linoleic acid or arachidonic acid concentrations, increased plasma mead acid concentrations, and/or elevated triene (eicosatrienoic acid with 3 double bonds, C20:3ω-9)-to-tetraene (arachidonic acid with 4 double bonds, C20:4ω-6) ratio > 0.2 (refer to specific laboratory normal ranges for the triene-to-tetraene ratio that may differ between laboratories). Plasma essential fatty acid profile should be regularly monitored (e.g., every 2 to 3 months) whenever intravenous lipid emulsion infusion or oral fat intake is restricted.

Clinical signs of essential fatty acid deficiency include dry flaky desquamating skin, poor wound healing, sparse hair growth, hair loss, eczematoid dermatosis of the face and neck, anemia, thrombocytopenia, and enlarged fatty liver. To prevent essential fatty acid deficiency, linoleic acid should provide a minimum of about 2% to 4% of total daily calorie intake. Practically, adult patients should be provided with 500 mL once weekly or 250 mL biweekly of 20% intravenous lipid emulsions to prevent essential fatty acid deficiency. In infants and children, an average daily dose of 0.5 to 1 g/kg/day of intravenous lipid emulsions is needed to prevent essential fatty acid deficiency. Due to their limited reserves and higher energy expenditure, preterm infants may develop biochemical essential fatty deficiency within 3 days of fat-free feeding.

HYPERCAPNIA

Hypercapnia describes the excess retention of carbon dioxide. This can occur with excess calorie and/or dextrose (or carbohydrates) intake that exceed the patient's metabolic capacity. Hypercapnia can lead to respiratory decompensation and may result in unsuccessful attempts to wean the patient from ventilator support. Metabolically, this may be reflected in increased respiratory quotient (RQ). The RQ describes the ratio of carbon dioxide production (VCO_2) relative to oxygen consumption (VO_2). A RQ > 1 indicates possible overfeeding with increased fat synthesis. Patients with compromised respiratory function are at greater risk for hypercapnia because of their limited alveolar reserve and less efficient carbon dioxide excretion. If a patient develops hypercapnia while receiving nutrition support, overfeeding should be rule out. The PN regimen should be revised to provide sufficient calories, yet minimize carbon dioxide production, by decreasing total calories and/or the dextrose load.

COMPLICATIONS OF OVERFEEDING

Excessive calorie administration (overfeeding) has detrimental consequences that affect the liver, pulmonary, and immunologic systems. Dextrose overfeeding may cause hyperglycemia, hepatic steatosis, and hypertriglyceridemia. Overfeeding from intravenous lipid emulsions can result in hypertriglyceridemia and congestion of the reticuloendothelial system, may affect pulmonary microcirculation, and causes respiratory compromise in neonates. Excess protein intake results in azotemia. Overall, overfeeding from macronutrients increases carbon dioxide production that causes respiratory compromise in patients with limited pulmonary reserve and prolongation of patient dependence on mechanical ventilation, causes liver toxicity (e.g., cholestasis, steatosis), and promotes excessive weight gain.

FLUID EXCESS

Excessive fluid infusion in the PN admixture can result in fluid overload to the patient. Signs and symptoms of fluid excess include rapid weight gain, peripheral edema, puffy eyelids, pulmonary edema, pleural effusion, ascites, elevated central venous pressure, and moist crackles. Fluid intake in the PN admixture should be adjusted based on the patient's clinical condition, especially in cases of decreased kidney function and congestive heart failure.

ELECTROLYTE ABNORMALITIES

PN should not be used to replace acute electrolyte deficiencies. Electrolytes in PN should be reduced as needed when the corresponding serum electrolyte concentrations are elevated. Acute renal and gastrointestinal electrolyte losses are best replaced via a separate infusion than PN.

Hyponatremia, Hypernatremia

Hyponatremia is the most common electrolyte abnormality in hospitalized patients. Hyponatremia is commonly caused by excessive hypotonic fluid intake and/or gastrointestinal losses of sodium-rich fluids (e.g., gastric suctioning, diarrhea, high ileostomy output). Hyponatremia is classified as isotonic, hypotonic, or hypertonic, and each type may require different treatment based on its etiology and severity. High serum glucose concentrations increase plasma osmolality to cause fluid shifting from the intracellular space into the plasma, resulting in hypertonic hyponatremia. Correction for serum sodium concentrations in the setting of hyperglycemia can be estimated as follows:

For each 100 mg/dL increase in serum glucose concentrations above 100 mg/dL, a 1.6 mEq/L is added to the measured serum sodium concentration.

In patients with hyponatremia related to sodium losses, sodium deficit is estimated using the following equation:

$$\text{Sodium deficit (mEq)} \simeq 0.6^a \times \text{body weight (kg)} \times (140 - \text{serum sodium})$$

[a]See below.

Hyponatremia should be corrected no faster than increasing serum sodium concentrations by a maximum of 12 mEq/L in 24 hours, to avoid potential precipitation of central pontine myelinolysis (CPM). Practically, about half of the deficit is replaced over the first 24 hours and the other half over the next 24 to 48 hours. Sodium in PN admixtures can be maximized to 154 mEq/L (normal saline equivalent) to reduce "free water" (hypotonic, low-sodium fluids) loading.

Hypernatremia is commonly the result of impaired water intake or relative water deficit. Hypernatremia is classified as isovolemic, hypovolemic, and hypervolemic, and treatment depends on the etiology and severity. Hypernatremia should be corrected no faster than decreasing serum sodium concentrations by a maximum of 12 mEq/L in 24 hours, to avoid potential precipitation of cerebral edema. Practically, about half of the deficit is replaced over the first 24 hours and the other half over the next 24 to 48 hours. When clinically indicated, additional sodium can be avoided in PN to increase "free water" delivery. Although amino acids may provide inherent sodium that cannot be avoided (Appendix H), these small amounts are relatively of little clinical impact in the overall spectrum of treating hypernatremia.

In patients with hypernatremia related to "free water" deficit, water deficit is estimated using the following equation:

$$\text{Free water deficit (L)} \simeq 0.6^a \times \text{body weight (kg)} \times [1 - (140/\text{serum sodium})]$$

[a]Percent of body weight that is water. This value is 0.6 for adult men, 0.5 for adult women, 0.55 for obese individuals, and 0.8 for infants.

Hypokalemia, Hypophosphatemia, Hypomagnesemia

Potassium, phosphorus, and magnesium share some common features: they are primarily excreted via the kidneys; their readily active components are mainly intracellular; and their requirements are increased during anabolism. Anabolism causes intracellular shift of potassium, phosphorus, and magnesium. Medications (e.g., loop and thiazide diuretics, amphotericin B, micafungin) cause renal potassium and magnesium losses. Alkalosis causes factitious hypokalemia by shifting potassium intracellularly. Electrolyte replacement is dictated by serum electrolyte concentrations with consideration of the patient's kidney function, acid-base status, electrolyte losses, and medication therapies. Coexisting hypomagnesemia and hypokalemia can lead to refractory hypokalemia, unless hypomagnesemia is corrected.

In infants, solubility limitations imposed on restricted calcium and phosphorus amounts in PN admixtures may result in hypocalcemia and hypophosphatemia. Hypomagnesemia is also encountered in newborn infants of diabetic mothers. Hypophosphatemia is common in preterm infants due to their low body phosphate stores and phosphorus wasting via their immature kidneys.

Hyperkalemia, Hyperphosphatemia, Hypermagnesemia

Potassium, phosphorus, and magnesium accumulate with decreased kidney function. During catabolism, these intracellular electrolytes are released from the intracellular space, which further increases their serum concentrations. Potassium-retaining medications (e.g., angiotensin-converting enzyme inhibitors, potassium-sparing diuretics, cyclosporine, tacrolimus) may cause hyperkalemia. Factitious hyperkalemia can result from acidosis that causes extracellular shift of potassium, or because of hemolyzed blood transfusion or from a heelstick blood draw.
In neonates, hypermagnesemia may result from maternal magnesium sulfate administration when treating preterm labor or pre-eclampsia. Serum

magnesium concentrations exceeding 2.8 mg/dL requires withholding magnesium in PN until serum magnesium concentrations return to normal.

Hypocalcemia

About 45% of serum calcium in bound to serum albumin. Hypocalcemia is commonly attributed to hypoalbuminemia, especially in malnourished patients. A one gram decrease in serum albumin results in approximately 0.8 mg decrease in serum calcium concentrations. Total serum calcium concentrations are estimated as follows:

Total serum calcium = measured serum calcium + 0.8 (4 − serum albumin)

For an accurate evaluation of serum calcium status, serum ionized calcium (free, active) concentrations should be measured when serum albumin concentrations are low. Alkalemia increases calcium binding to serum albumin and acidemia decreases calcium binding to serum albumin, which will affect serum ionized calcium concentrations.

Hypercalcemia

Hypercalcemia is rarely caused by excess calcium in PN. Common causes of hypercalcemia are malignancies, hyperparathyroidism, and immobilization. Calcium and phosphorus should be omitted from PN when the product of serum calcium and phosphorus concentrations exceeds 60 mg^2/dL^2 in order to avoid metastatic calcification.

ACID-BASE DISORDERS

Acid-base disorders are mainly caused by the patient's underlying disease(s) and clinical conditions(s). Although PN is rarely a cause of acid-base disorders, providing unbalanced or excessive chloride and acetate in PN can alter the patient's acid-base balance. Hyperchloremic acidosis may result from large and rapid infusion of normal saline fluids. Hyperchloremic acidosis can also be caused by significant bicarbonate losses from the intestines or kidneys (subsequently causing chloride retention) and renal tubular acidosis (proximal, distal). In infants and children, excessive chloride amounts exceeding 6 mEq/kg/day increase the risk for metabolic acidosis. Excessive protein intake in neonates, especially preterm infants, may also cause metabolic acidosis. In adults, serum chloride concentrations exceeding 130 mEq/L may result in metabolic acidosis. Acetate in vivo is converted to bicarbonate. Excessive acetate in PN causes excess alkali load that may result in metabolic alkalosis with possible hypoventilation as a compensatory response in severe cases or highly susceptible patients. Metabolic alkalosis may be worsened in patients with risk factors for contraction alkalosis (e.g., high-dose loop or thiazide diuretics, vomiting, high gastric fluid suctioning) or with concurrent administration of oral or intravenous bicarbonate or Lactated

Ringers fluids (lactate converted to bicarbonate). A normal chloride-to-acetate ratio in PN is 1.5-to-1. Adjustments to the amounts of chloride and acetate in PN should be guided by the patient's acid-base and clinical status. Regular monitoring of serum electrolytes (especially potassium) and appropriate electrolyte supplementation are indicated with acid-base imbalances, especially in patients with kidney, liver, or pulmonary diseases.

REFEEDING SYNDROME

Refeeding syndrome is characterized by fluid and electrolyte imbalances, glucose intolerance, and vitamin deficiencies that occur in malnourished patients who are refed after chronic starvation and significant weight loss. During starvation, there is an increase in total body water, sodium retention, and depletion of potassium, magnesium, phosphorus, and vitamin stores. The size and function of the heart, kidneys, and intestines are decreased. Individuals who are refed orally, enterally, or parenterally after severe weight loss are at risk for refeeding syndrome. Individuals at risk for refeeding syndrome include those with anorexia nervosa, prolonged fasting, chronic alcoholism, chronic malnutrition, significant weight loss, and those receiving prolonged intravenous hydration.

Complications of refeeding may affect the cardiac, pulmonary, hematologic, and neuromuscular systems. Severe cases of refeeding have resulted in cardiac failure, seizures, and death. The introduction of carbohydrates increases insulin secretion and the demand for phosphorylated intermediates in glycolysis (e.g., ATP, 2,3-DPG), and causes intracellular shift of potassium, phosphorus, and magnesium. In combination with preexisting low total body stores of potassium, phosphorus, and magnesium, this results in hypophosphatemia, hypokalemia, and hypomagnesemia. Intracellular phosphates are required for generation of high-energy phosphate bonds. Profound phosphorus depletion may lead to acute cardiopulmonary decompensation and possible death. Phosphate supplementation (as sodium or potassium phosphate) at doses up to 1 mmol/kg is necessary to treat severe hypophosphatemia in patients with normal kidney function.

Clinicians should identify patients at risk for refeeding and take steps to prevent refeeding syndrome. Aggressive electrolyte supplementation including potassium, phosphate, and magnesium before and during nutrient delivery is required, along with vitamin supplementation and supportive care. A rule of thumb for initiating nutrition in patients at risk for refeeding syndrome is to start low and advance slowly to nutritional goal. Nutrition should begin at about 25% of nutrition requirements and advanced gradually to nutritional goal over the next 3 to 5 days. Serum potassium, magnesium, and phosphorus concentrations should be monitored twice daily during the first few days of nutrition initiation, and electrolytes should be supplemented as needed. Because water-soluble vitamin deficiencies can rapidly occur, oral or intravenous multivitamin supplementation should be provided in addition to thiamine (e.g., 100 mg/day for adults) and folic acid (e.g., 1 mg/day for adults) for the first 7 days.

TRACE ELEMENTS ABNORMALITIES

Trace element imbalances occur in the setting of disease states or when abnormal trace element intake and losses occur. Monitoring trace element status is challenging because serum trace element concentrations may not reflect total body or tissue trace element stores. Further, stress causes redistribution of trace elements in the liver and tissues and increases urinary trace element excretion (e.g., zinc, selenium) without necessarily indicating body trace element depletion or deficiency. Although no specific guidelines are available for the frequency of monitoring trace element status, a reasonable schedule is to monitor serum trace element concentrations every 3 months at first following the initiation of PN therapy or whenever a change is made to trace element supplementation, and every 6 to 12 months thereafter in stable patients.

Manganese

Manganese accumulation occurs in patients with cholestatic liver disease due to the obstruction of bile flow, the main route for manganese excretion. Even in the absence of cholestasis, long-term PN-dependent patients may have elevated serum manganese concentrations, possibly because current recommendations for daily manganese supplementation in PN exceed the actual requirements. Neurotoxicity (e.g., tremor, gait, mask-like face, muscle rigidity, headache, confusion, somnolence, weakness) has been reported with manganese accumulation in cholestatic patients receiving long-term PN containing manganese. Magnetic resonance imaging (MRI) has shown manganese deposits in the basal ganglia of PN-dependent patients with high serum manganese concentrations. Neurological symptoms are reversible when manganese is withheld from PN. Because bile flow cannot be easily measured, it is common practice to restrict manganese from PN when serum direct bilirubin concentrations exceed 2 mg/dL, and when serum manganese concentrations are elevated or manganese toxicity is suspected.

Copper

Copper accumulation may occur in patients with cholestasis due to the obstruction of bile flow, the main route for copper excretion. Asymptomatic increases in serum copper concentrations and liver copper accumulation have been reported in PN patients with cholestasis. However, elimination of copper from the PN of cholestatic patients has resulted in copper deficiency. Clinical signs and symptoms of copper deficiency include pancytopenia, hypochromic microcytic anemia, leukopenia, osteopenia, depigmentation of hair and skin, and neurologic disturbances. Pancytopenia from copper deficiency occurred within 6 weeks to 15 months after copper was omitted form PN. Pancytopenia in reported cases of copper deficiency resulted in patient deaths or was reversed in other cases following copper supplementation. It is common practice to restrict copper from PN in patients with serum direct bilirubin concentrations exceeding 2 mg/dL. However, this threshold does not reflect a complete biliary obstruction, and a lower rate of biliary copper elimination may still occur. When copper is restricted from PN, serum copper concentrations should be measured regularly (e.g., every 1 month following copper restriction, and less frequently thereafter) to avoid copper deficiency.

Zinc

Zinc is mainly excreted in the intestines and urinary zinc losses are increased in patients under metabolic stress (e.g., critical illness). Fecal zinc losses are increased in patients with severe diarrhea, malabsorption syndromes (e.g., short bowel syndrome), and high-output fluid losses from ileostomy and enterocutaneous fistulae. Severe thermal injury (burns) and trauma patients may also have increased zinc losses. Severe zinc deficiency may cause growth retardation in children, hypogonadism, poor wound healing, infertility, dermatitis, alopecia, impaired immunity, glossitis and dysgeusia. Empiric intravenous zinc supplementation at 15 mg/day has been used in adult patients with severe diarrhea or with high-output ileostomy or enterocutaneous fistulae. Because zinc enhances wound healing, adult patients with severe thermal injury or large wounds may require daily supplementation of oral zinc sulfate at an oral dose of 220 mg or a total of 15 mg of elemental zinc in PN. In infants and children, empiric adjustments of zinc amounts in PN can be achieved by empiric increases or decreases (e.g., 25%, 50%) of zinc supplements in or outside the PN admixture, guided by regular monitoring of serum zinc concentrations.

Selenium

Selenium is a cofactor of glutathione peroxidase, a major intracellular antioxidant enzyme. Selenium is primarily eliminated via the kidneys. However, significant selenium losses occur in patients with severe diarrhea or malabsorption syndromes (e.g., short bowel syndrome), and high-output fluid losses from ileostomy and enterocutaneous fistulae. Selenium supplementation between 90 and 150 mcg/day may be necessary to correct or maintain normal serum selenium concentrations in these patients. Critically ill patients may show decreased serum selenium concentrations and increased urinary selenium losses. However, the clinical significance of these changes is unknown. Although unlikely to occur in patients receiving PN, severe selenium deficiency manifests in painful muscle weakness, cardiomyopathy, and erythrocyte macrocytsosis. In patients who receive PN without selenium supplementation, serum selenium concentrations are decreased along with decreased glutathione peroxidase activity. The clinical consequences of reduced glutathione peroxidase activity are unknown. The optimal selenium dose to correct deficiency is unknown. Empiric adjustments to selenium amounts in PN can be achieved by increases or decreases (e.g., 25%, 50%) of selenium supplementation in or outside the PN admixture, guided by regular monitoring of serum selenium concentrations.

LIVER COMPLICATIONS

Transient elevation of liver function tests without any consistent liver pathological changes have been reported within a few weeks after PN initiation, but these abnormalities generally resolve after PN is stopped. Most common liver complications associated with PN include cholestasis, steatosis, and cholelithiasis.

Cholestasis

PN-associated cholestasis (PNAC) is the most common and life-threatening liver toxicity associated with PN. Although PNAC is usually a complication of chronic PN-dependence, it can occur in infants within 1 to 2 weeks of PN initiation. The etiology of PNAC is multifactorial. Factors that correlate with PNAC include long-term PN, lack of oral or enteral feeding for intestinal stimulation, excessive calorie administration (overfeeding), recurrent sepsis, significant intestinal resection (e.g., short bowel syndrome), and bacterial translocation.

The hallmarks of the clinical presentation of PNAC include jaundice, pruritus, and elevated serum conjugated bilirubin concentrations (exceeding 2 mg/dL). Physiologically, PNAC is associated with decreased canalicular bile flow and jaundice. Liver histopathology shows periportal inflammation, bile duct proliferation, intralobular cholestasis, bile plugging, fibrosis, cirrhosis, and steatosis that appear at various stages. Severe PNAC can lead to progressive liver failure and death. However, PNAC can be reversible if PN is discontinued before the progression to end-stage liver disease. Serum biliribun concentrations may take as long as 3 months to return to normal following PN discontinuation. Patients with severe PNAC should be evaluated for possible isolated bowel or combined liver and bowel transplantation.

Clinical measures to avoid or reduce the risk of PNAC include optimizing calorie intake and avoiding overfeeding; early initiation of oral or enteral nutrition to maintain gut motility and integrity; limiting intravenous lipid emulsion infusion to once or twice weekly to a minimum dose to prevent essential fatty acid deficiency; cyclic infusion of PN over less than 24 hours to avoid continuous compulsive nutrient loading on the liver; preventing and prompt treatment of infections (e.g., catheter-related bloodstream infections); and treatment of bacterial overgrowth preferably by alternating non-absorbable antimicrobials (e.g., oral gentamicin, neomycin), or the use of other antimicrobials when indicated (e.g., metronidazole, ciprofloxacin).

At the earliest signs of increased serum direct bilirubin or gamma-glutamyl transpeptidase (GGT) concentrations, treatment with ursodeoxycholic acid (ursodiol) 10 to 15 mg/kg/day in adults and 10 to 30 mg/kg/day in children divided in 2 to 3 doses has shown to improve the biochemical signs (i.e., serum bilirubin and transaminases concentrations) and clinical symptoms (e.g., jaundice, hepatosplenomegaly) of PNAC. However, ursodiol long-term effects on PNAC and in preventing progression to end-stage liver disease are unknown. Further, ursodiol at recommended doses, especially in patients with malabsorption and with terminal ileal and/or jejunal resections (e.g., short bowel syndrome), may not consistently achieve therapeutic effects. Higher ursodiol doses may cause or aggravate diarrhea (bile-induced diarrhea). Treatment with intravenous cholecystokinin-octapeptide (sincalide) 0.04 mcg/kg twice daily to stimulate gallbladder contraction and bile flow failed to prevent PNAC or improve serum conjugated bilirubin concentrations, and is not recommended for treating or preventing PNAC.

There is increased interest in the use of fish oil-based intravenous lipid emulsions containing primarily omega-3 fatty acids in patients with PNAC. Soybean oil-based intravenous lipid emulsions contain primarily omega-6 fatty acids that are proinflammatory, and also contain phytosterols, both believed to contribute to liver injury in PN patients. Preliminary data in infants have shown that PNAC can be potentially reversed with the use of fish oil-based intravenous lipids (dose 1 g/kg/day) instead of soybean/safflower oil-based lipid emulsions. Data from large prospective randomized clinical studies are needed to further assess the efficacy of fish oil-based intravenous lipid emulsions in preventing PNAC. Fish oil-based intravenous lipid emulsions are not currently available on the US market.

Steatosis

Hepatic steatosis or fatty liver describes fat (e.g., triglycerides, cholesterol esters) accumulation in the hepatocytes as a result of imbalance between liver fat secretion and synthesis. Steatohepatitis (non-alcoholic) is a rare complication associated with PN therapy and is characterized by advanced liver disease with hepatic inflammation that may rapidly progress to cirrhosis.

Hepatic steatosis in PN patients results from dextrose (*de novo* lipogenesis presumably due to increased insulin-to-glucagon ratio) or lipid overfeeding. The role of certain nutrient deficiencies such as carnitine, choline, and essential fatty acids in predisposing to hepatic steatosis is less clear. Patients with hepatic steatosis are usually asymptomatic, but hepatomegaly, malaise, and abdominal discomfort may be present and should prompt further patient evaluation. Fat-overload syndrome (hypertriglyceridemia, fever, hepatosplenomegaly, coagulopathy, multiorgan dysfunction) was reported with high intravenous lipid emulsion doses exceeding 4 g/kg/day, which far exceeded the maximum recommended intravenous lipid doses of 1 g/kg/day in adults and 3 g/kg/day in children.

Hepatic steatosis is usually reversible when a portion of dextrose is replaced with lipid calories. It is also important to avoid overfeeding and provide a balanced PN regimen (total daily calories of 20% to 30% from intravenous lipid emulsions, 50% to 60% from dextrose, and 10% to 20% from amino acids).

Cholelithiasis

Cholelithiasis (gallstones) in PN patients is caused by decreased gallbladder contractility in the absence of oral or enteral feeding. During fasting, cholecystokinin (CCK) secretion in the duodenum is absent leading to decreased gallbladder contractility. This causes the bile to accumulate in the biliary tract which favors cholesterol gallstone formation and calcium bilirubinate precipitation (i.e., sludge).

Patients with short bowel syndrome are at high risk for cholelithiasis due to their disrupted enterohepatic cycling (when terminal ileum is resected), impaired bile flow (because of fasting), and canalicular accumulation of toxic bile (e.g., lithocholic acid).

Cholelithiasis can best be prevented by early oral or enteral nutrition to stimulate CCK secretion, gallbladder emptying, and intestinal motility. Cholecystectomy may be indicated in symptomatic patients with cholecystitis or choledocholithiasis. Injections of cholecystokinin-octapeptide to induce gallbladder contractions have not shown to prevent PN-associated cholelithiasis.

METABOLIC BONE DISEASE

Metabolic bone disease associated with PN may present as osteomalacia (soft bones, with defective bone mineralization and excess osteoid accumulation), osteopenia (low bone mass with decreased bone mineralization) and/or osteoporosis (porous bones with decreased total bone mass). About 40% to 100% of PN-dependent patients may have some degree of bone demineralization (e.g., in spine, hip, femoral, neck). Although metabolic bone disease in adult patients occurs mostly during chronic PN therapy, infants and children may develop bone mineral defects much earlier. Signs and symptoms of metabolic bone disease include bone pain, pathologic bone fractures, elevated serum alkaline phosphatase, increased serum parathyroid hormone (PTH) concentrations (secondary hyperparathyroidism), hypercalciuria, and a washed-out demineralized bone appearance on X-ray.

Etiologies of metabolic bone disease in PN patients include calcium and phosphorus deficiencies due to solubility limitation in PN admixtures, and aluminum toxicity. Aluminum contamination of PN admixtures is mostly from calcium and phosphate salts, trace elements, and heparin additives. Preterm infants and patients with renal insufficiency are at highest risk for aluminum accumulation. Aluminum toxicity may cause osteomalacia, neurologic toxicity, and hypochromic microcytic anemia. Aluminum effects on the bones are possibly via its effects on impairing calcium bone fixation, inhibiting the conversion of the intermediate 25-hydroxyvitamin D metabolite to the active 1, 25-dihydroxyvitamin D, and by reducing PTH synthesis.

The Food and Drug Administration (FDA) has issued rules and warnings about aluminum contamination of parenteral products. The FDA rule, issued in the year 2000, required that large-volume parenteral products (amino acids, dextrose, intravenous lipid emulsions, sterile water) used in compounding PN admixtures must contain no more than 25 micrograms/L of aluminum. Small volume parenteral products (parenteral electrolyte, vitamins, and trace element products) should be labeled with the maximum aluminum content at expiration. Because toxic aluminum effects occur at the microgram levels, the FDA defined a safe upper limit for parenteral aluminum intake at 5 mcg/kg/day, although tissue aluminum loading may still occur at this level, especially in patients with renal insufficiency and premature kidney function.

The prevention and treatment of metabolic bone disease in PN patients relies mostly on maximizing calcium and phosphorus intake, avoiding vitamin D deficiency, and minimizing exposure to aluminum. PN-dependent patients would benefit from regular low-intensity exercise to improve their lumbar spine bone density. Products with the lowest aluminum content should be used in compounding PN admixtures. However, it remains difficult to meet the FDA safety limit for aluminum loading in the daily PN formulation. Bisphosphonates (e.g., pamidronate, clodronate) inhibit osteoclast-mediated bone resorption and have been reported to possibly improve the signs and symptoms of metabolic bone disease in PN-dependent patients. However, the role of bisphosphonates in PN patients with metabolic bone disease requires further studies.

Routine monitoring of serum vitamin D, calcium, phosphorus, and PTH concentrations is recommended, and bone density measurements every 1 to 2 years are suggested in PN-dependent patients for early detection of metabolic bone disease whenever it occurs.

XIII. INFECTIOUS COMPLICATIONS ASSOCIATED WITH PARENTERAL NUTRITION

CATHETER-RELATED BLOODSTREAM INFECTIONS

Catheter-related bloodstream infections (CRBSI) in patients receiving parenteral nutrition (PN) are the most common complications associated with central venous access device(s) (VAD) used for central PN infusion. CRBSI are associated with increased patient morbidity and mortality, hospitalization and prolonged hospital stay, and increased healthcare costs.

Microorganisms frequently associated with CRBSI include *Staphylococcus epidermidis*, *Staphylococcus aureus*, *Enterococci*, *Escherichia coli*, *Klebsiella*, *Enterobacter*, and *Candida* species.

Factors that increase the risk of CRBSI include duration of catheterization, use of VAD for multiple treatment purposes (e.g., chemotherapy, blood drawing, blood product administration, PN, medication administration, venous pressure reading, catheter clot extraction), duration of PN therapy, prematurity (immature immune system), lower extremity VAD insertion site (e.g., femoral), and the use of multiple-lumen VAD (versus single-lumen VAD).

Protective and preventive measures can be undertaken to prevent CRBSI, including staff education and training on infection control practices (e.g., hand hygiene, aseptic techniques), using maximum barrier precautions during VAD insertion (e.g., wearing gloves, gown, mask, cap, using large drape), and using topical skin antiseptics (e.g., chlorhexidine 2%). Sterile techniques should be followed using occlusive dressings after VAD insertion to reduce bacterial colonization at the VAD insertion site and avoid the risk of systemic infections. The use of VAD for multiple treatment purposes should be kept to a minimum. Ideally, infected VAD should be replaced, but sometimes technical and anatomical issues may limit available insertion sites. Guidelines for the diagnosis and management of CRBSIs have been published by the Infectious Diseases Society of America (IDSA) (Mermel LA, Allon M, Bouza E, et al. Clinical practice guidelines for the diagnosis and management of intravascular catheter-related infection: 2009 update by the Infectious Diseases Society of America. Clin Infect Dis 2009;49:1-45).

Clinical Presentation of Catheter-Related Bloodstream Infections

Localized infections at the VAD insertion site (i.e., exit site infection) may include erythema, induration, tenderness, and purulent exudates within 2 cm of the skin at the exit site, in the absence of bloodstream infection. Tunnel infections present with symptoms similar to the exit site infection, but extend beyond 2 cm of the skin at the exit site. Pocket infections are confined to implanted catheters and may present with erythema and necrosis of the skin over the port reservoir or with purulent exudates in the subcutaneous pocket.

Infusion-related sepsis should be suspected if the following signs and symptoms occur within 1 to 2 hours after administration of a new PN admixture: fever, chills, headache, hypotension, flushing, nausea, vomiting, malaise, oliguria, hyperglycemia, or general deterioration in patient's clinical condition. If the PN admixture itself is suspected as the source of infection, the suspected PN admixture should be stopped, the entire PN infusion set with a sterile needle capping the distal tubing and the entire unused portion of the bag or bottle should be sent to the Microbiology Laboratory for aerobic, anaerobic, and fungi cultures. New PN admixture and intravenous tubing should be used or an appropriate dextrose in water replacement solution should be infused until the next PN admixture becomes available.

CONSIDERATIONS FOR PARENTERAL NUTIRITION INFUSION IN FEBRILE PATIENTS

The source of fever should be investigated prior to PN initiation. PN should not be initiated during the early stages of an uncontrolled infection, particularly during recurrent bacteremia or sepsis.

Workup Protocol of Possible Vascular Access Device Sepsis

1. Investigate all possible sources of infection (e.g., lungs, genitourinary, abdomen, wounds, bloodstream). VAD should not be routinely replaced simply to prevent CRBSI
2. If there is evidence of infection such as purulence, inflammation, or phlebitis at the VAD exit site, the VAD should be removed and replaced with a new insertion site
3. If no other septic source is found after 24 hours, the VAD should best be removed. The benefits of VAD replacement must be weighed against the risk of complications from VAD insertion in each patient
4. If the VAD is being replaced because of suspected infection, the new VAD should be inserted at new site. The risks and benefits of exchange over a guidewire in this situation must be assessed on an individual basis. Exchanging the VAD over a guidewire increases the risk of bloodstream infection in case of exit-site infection
5. Draw quantitative blood cultures (aerobes and anaerobes) through the VAD and from a peripheral venous site. If blood culture returns positive, the VAD should be removed. The VAD tip should also be cultured after VAD removal
6. To culture the VAD, prepare the skin, remove the VAD, cut off a one-inch piece at the VAD tip with sterile scissors and place into a sterile container, send the VAD sample to the Microbiology Laboratory for aerobic, anaerobic, and fungi cultures

7. If a VAD is removed because of suspected bacteremia and it must be replaced, wait for at least 24 hours after appropriate antibiotic therapy is begun or after three successive negative blood cultures, and reinsert the VAD at a different site
8. To decrease the likelihood of VAD-related sepsis, the infusion set for PN admixtures without intravenous lipid emulsions must be replaced every 96 hours. The infusion set for intravenous lipid emulsions must be replaced every 24 hours
9. Do not to use the VAD lumens for other than PN. However, the PN admixture may be infused through a VAD lumen that was used for other purposes prior to PN initiation. Once the PN infusion is discontinued, the VAD lumen may again be used for other treatment purposes

Indications for Vascular Access Device Removal

- Catheter tunnel infection
- VAD exit-site infection
- Persistent fever with no other source of infection
- Severe sepsis or septic shock
- Pulmonary embolization or infective endocarditis
- Ongoing bacteremia after 48 to 72 hours following antimicrobial therapy
- Relapse of infection after discontinuation of antimicrobial therapy
- CRBSI due to yeasts (*Candida* species), other fungi, and mycobacteria pathogens
- CRBSI due to gram negative organisms (e.g., *Escherichia coli*, *Klebsiella* species, *Pseudomonas* species)
- CRBSI due to *Staphylococcus aureus*. *Staphylococcus aureus* adheres to the catheter surface by surface receptors that involve specific host protein interactions. Serious complications may also arise with *Staphylococcus aureus* infections such as septic thrombosis, endocarditits, severe sepsis, or deep-seated infections. Low cure rate, high risk of relapse, and increased mortality may occur if the VAD is not removed
- CRBSI due to *Bacillus* or *Corynebacterium* species
- Some organisms including *Staphylococcus aureus*, *Bacillus* species, *Pseudomonas* species, and others form an exopolysaccharide biofilm (slime) that clings tenaciously to the surface of the VAD and protects them from phagocytic cells, antibodies, and antibiotics, usually precluding eradication of infection without device removal
- Consultation with an infectious diseases specialist may be indicated if the VAD cannot be removed

Refer to the following internal website for Infection Control policies on central and arterial vascular access devices: http://www.med.umich.edu/i/ice/.

ANTIBIOTIC LOCK TECHNIQUE

The antibiotic lock technique describes the concept of instilling high concentrations of antimicrobials inside the VAD lumen to treat or prevent intraluminal VAD infections. This technique is reserved to infections confined to the VAD lumen in the absence of sepsis or distant infectious sites. It is usually used in combination with or following a course of systemic antibiotic therapy. The antibiotic lock technique is mainly used for long-term home PN-dependent patients who frequently develop VAD-related infections and who present anatomical difficulties in replacing the VAD. Advantages of the antibiotic lock technique include sterilization of the VAD lumen, avoidance of VAD removal, and avoidance of antimicrobials systemic side effects. Prior to accessing the VAD, the antibiotic lock should be withdrawn and discarded to prevent antibiotic resistance.

The types of antimicrobials used depend on the type and sensitivity of the cultured microorganisms. A concentrated antimicrobial solution with a volume of approximately 1 to 4 mL (depending on VAD type) is allowed to dwell in the VAD between PN infusions. The antimicrobial solution is withdrawn from the VAD, and the VAD is then flushed with normal saline before PN is infused. Examples of parenteral antibiotic regimen used for the VAD antibiotic lock therapy include Vancomycin (0.025 mg/mL), Gentamicin (0.02 mg/mL), Cefazolin (0.5 mg/mL), or Linezolid (1.8 mg/mL); all can individually be combined with heparin 10 units/mL. The Infectious Disease service should be consulted for appropriate indication and dosing.

ETHANOL LOCK TECHNIQUE

Similar to antibiotic locks, ethanol lock consists of instilling the VAD lumen with a 70% ethanol lock solution to treat and prevent CRBSI. The ethanol lock therapy is used for permanent silicone central VAD, including central tunneled VAD (e.g., Broviac®, Hickman®) and implanted ports ≥ 6.6 French that are placed in the University of Michigan, C.S. Mott Children's Hospital operating room. Heparin and citrate are incompatible with ethanol and should not be mixed or infused simultaneously.

The ethanol lock therapy avoids antibiotic resistance and its efficacy is independent of the sensitivity results of the offending microorganisms. To be effective, the ethanol lock solution must dwell into the VAD lumen for a minimum of 2 hours. For long-term PN patients, this can be accomplished during the time when the PN admixture is not infusing.

Several precautions should be taken when using the ethanol lock therapy
- Ethanol lock therapy can only be used in silicone VAD, and should not be used in polyurethane VAD
- The VAD volume must be calculated prior to instillation (Chapter XIX, Table 3)

- Instill 0.1 to 0.7 mL of the 70% ethanol (depending on the VAD internal volume), remove, and flush before and after instillation with 5 mL of normal saline
- Label the VAD indicating that ethanol has been instilled
- If ethanol cannot be aspirated and must be infused, blood alcohol level should not exceed 0.04
- Side effects may include tiredness, headaches, dizziness, nausea, and light-headedness

Refer to the following internal website for the Ethanol Lock Therapy
in C.S. Mott Children's Hospital policy (07-01-018)
http://www.med.umich.edu/i/policies/umh/07-01-018.html.

XIV. ENTERAL NUTRITION ORDERING AND ADMINISTRATION FOR ADULT PATIENTS

ORDERING ENTERAL NUTRITION

Enteral nutrition (EN) orders are placed in CareLink (Computerized Prescriber Order Entry, CPOE). Choices of EN formulas and enteral feeding rates are outlined in CareLink.

ADMINISTRATION MODES OF ENTERAL NUTRITION

The site of tube feeding and EN delivery method are often determined by the patient's underlying diseases and gastrointestinal surgeries. Gastric feeding is most physiologic and is the preferred route for EN delivery. In some patients with delayed gastric emptying or other gastric abnormalities, the optimal site of tube feeding is the duodenum or jejunum.

Continuous Enteral Nutrition

Continuous gastric and small intestine feedings provide daily calorie and protein requirements at a constant rate over 24 hours, and are generally delivered using an infusion pump. Generally, continuous feedings are initiated at full strength of 30 mL/hr for 6 hours, and advanced by 25 mL/hr every 6 hours to nutritional goal. Feedings can also be cycled down to run over 12 hours. Continuous gastric feeding is indicated for ventilator-dependent critically ill patients and those with malabsorption syndromes. Duodenal and jejunal feedings are best tolerated by continuous feeding. It is common practice to refer to "trophic feedings" in adult patients as continuous administration of EN at a steady rate of 10 mL/hr. This minimal rate is to test the gastrointestinal tolerance to EN, and theoretically to maintain a relative intestinal functionality, integrity, blood flow, hormone release, enzyme activity, gut immunity, and microbial flora. Although these are the desired benefits of "trophic feedings", there is no high-quality evidence to indicate that the projected benefits are necessarily achieved at this EN administration rate.

Intermittent Enteral Nutrition

Intermittent gastric EN is indicated for patients who require supplementation of oral nutrition. Intermittent feedings provide protein and calorie requirements at prescribed intervals and can only be used in patients with a gastric feeding tube. Typically, a large volume of EN formula is administered over 1 hour (range of 20 minutes to 2 hours) every 2 to 4 hours by gravity. Intermittent feedings should be initiated with a small amount of EN formula, and gradually increased to goal over 1 to 2 days in the hospital. Generally, 120 mL is given for the first feeding, 240 mL for the next two feedings, and

360 mL for the next three feedings, up to 480 mL per feeding, until the nutritional goal is reached. Although there is no exact rate at which intermittent feedings should be administered, the delivery rate can be altered by adjusting the clamp on the gravity feeding bag.

NASOENTERIC FEEDING TUBE PLACEMENT

Equipment

- Size 8 or 12 French tube and stylet
- Exam gloves
- Lubricant (petroleum jelly)
- Glass of water and a straw, or ice chips
- Emesis basin
- Tape

Procedure

1. Provide privacy
2. Explain procedure and its purpose
3. Elevate the head of bed at least 45 degrees with neck flexed slightly, if possible
4. Insert stylet into feeding tube and lock in place
5. Inspect nares and determine optimal patency by having the patient breathe through one nostril while the other is temporarily occluded
6. Estimate approximate distance for placement into the stomach by measuring the length from the tip of the nose to the ear lobe, and then from the ear lobe to the xyphoid process. Add 50 cm to this length if small bowel placement is desired. Mark either gastric or small bowel endpoint with permanent ink
7. Lubricate the end of the feeding tube with petroleum jelly and pass it posteriorly. If the patient is able, ask the patient to swallow water to facilitate passage of the tube
8. Advance the tube to the 25 cm mark, stopping at any point if resistance is met. Listen to the end of the tube for any signs of air movement. If air flow is evident or the patient begins coughing or resistance is met when trying to advance the tube, withdraw the tube and allow the patient to rest before re-attempting. If no air flow or resistance is evident, continue to advance the tube down the esophagus with the head in a neutral position until the gastric endpoint is reached. Proceed to step "e" (below) if gastric placement is the goal
9. If tube placement into the small bowel is necessary
   a. Advance the tube until subtle resistance is felt when the tip is at the pylorus
   b. Continue to gently advance the tip a short distance and hold against the pylorus

c. Continue to hold pressure on the tube; a "give" will be felt once the pylorus relaxes and the tube passes into the duodenum (this may take 10 to 20 minutes with additional sips of water)
d. Gently advance the tube as it is pulled by duodenal motility until endpoint is reached
e. Confirm proper tube placement by a "low upright" chest X-ray

ADMINISTRATION PROCEDURES OF CONTINUOUS ENTERAL NUTRITION

Equipment

- EN formula
- Feeding bag with tubing
- Infusion pump
- Graduated container
- Catheter tip 60 mL syringe
- 2-inch tape
- Water

Procedure

1. Explain procedure to the patient
2. Elevate the head of bed at 30 to 45 degrees
3. Wash hands
4. Wipe off the top of the EN formula cans and allow the EN formula to warm to room temperature
5. Clamp the feeding bag tubing. Shake the EN cans. Measure an 8-hour volume in the graduated container and pour into the feeding bag. Close lid. Cover any unused portion of the EN formula, label with date and time, and place in refrigerator
6. Hang the feeding bag on the intravenous pole. Squeeze the drip chamber until half full. Open the feeding bag clamp and prime the tubing. Re-clamp the feeding bag
7. Place the tubing into the infusion pump according to manufacturer's directions
8. Remove the cap from the patient's tube and flush with 30 to 50 mL water using a 60 mL syringe. Skip to step "10" if it is small intestine feeding tube
9. For gastric feedings, gently aspirate contents using a 60 mL syringe
    a. If gastric residual volumes (GRV) are greater than twice the hourly feeding rate, refeed the aspirate up to 200 mL into the stomach, flush with 30 mL of water, and clamp the feeding tube. Recheck the GRV after one hour, and if still greater than twice the hourly feeding rate, notify the physician

b. If GRV are lesser than twice the hourly rate, refeed the aspirate, flush the feeding tube with 30 to 50 mL of water, and proceed with tube feeding administration

10. Attach the feeding bag tubing to the patient's feeding tube. Reinforce the connection with tape and label "TF" for "tube feeding"
11. Open the clamp on the feeding bag and administer the EN formula at the prescribed rate
12. After the feeding is administered, disconnect the tubing and flush the feeding tube with 60 mL of water. Recap the feeding tube
13. Document the type and amount of EN formula, amount of water given, and the patient's tolerance

ADMINISTRATION PROCEDURES OF INTERMITTENT ENTERAL NUTRITION

Equipment

- Formula
- Gravity feeding bag with tubing
- 60 mL catheter tip syringe
- 2-inch tape
- Graduated container
- Water

Procedure

1. Explain procedure to the patient. Provide a schedule of subsequent feedings
2. Elevate the head of bed at 30 to 45 degrees during feeding
3. Wash hands
4. Wipe off the top of the EN formula cans and allow the EN formula to warm to room temperature
5. Clamp the feeding bag tubing. Shake the formula cans. Measure the prescribed EN formula volume in the graduated container and pour into the feeding bag. Close lid. Cover any unused portion of the EN formula, label with date and time, and place in refrigerator
6. Hang the feeding bag on an intravenous pole that has been raised approximately 12 to 18 inches above the patient's abdomen
7. Squeeze the drip chamber half full. Open the feeding bag clamp and prime the tubing. Re-clamp the feeding bag tubing
8. Remove the cap from the patient's tube and flush with 30 mL of water. Skip to step "10" if it is small intestine feeding tube
9. Using the 60 mL syringe, gently aspirate gastrointestinal contents:
    a. If GRV are greater than twice the hourly feeding rate, refeed the aspirate up to 200 mL into the stomach, flush with 30 mL water, and

re-clamp the tube. Recheck GRV after one hour, and if still greater than twice the hourly rate, notify the physician
   b. If GRV are lesser than twice the hourly feeding rate, refeed residuals, flush tube with 30 to 50 mL of water, and continue with tube feeding administration
10. Attach feeding bag tubing to patient's tube. Reinforce the connection with a piece of tape and label "TF" for "tube feeding"
11. Open the clamp on the feeding bag and slowly administer the EN formula at the prescribed rate (usually 240 to 360 mL over 40 to 60 minutes)
12. After the feeding is administered, disconnect the tubing, and flush the feeding tube with 60 mL of water. Recap the feeding tube
13. Keep the head of bed elevated for 30 to 45 minutes after feeding is complete
14. Rinse the feeding bag and tubing with warm water. Close the bag lid
15. Document the GRV, the time feeding started and ended, the type and amount of EN formula administered, the amount of water given, and the patient's tolerance

HANG TIME OF ENTERAL NUTRITION FORMULAS

To reduce microbial contamination and infectious risk, the maximum hang time of full-strength EN formulas is 8 hours. Reconstituted EN formulas have a shorter hang time of 4 hours. If a modular (e.g., protein module, ProMod[®]; MCT oil; glucose polymers, Moducal[®]; fat/safflower oil, Microlipid[®]) is added to the original EN formula, the maximum hang time of the final formula is 4 hours.

XV. PARENTERAL NUTRITION ORDERING, COMPOUNDING, AND ADMINISTRATION

The Institute for Safe Medical Practices (ISMP) lists parenteral nutrition (PN) admixtures under the class/category of high-alert medications. High-alert medications are described by the ISMP as "drugs that bear a heightened risk of causing significant patient harm when they are used in error. Although mistakes may or may not be more common with these drugs, the consequences of an error are clearly more devastating to patients." Policies and procedures (e.g., electronic prescriber order entry; standardizing ordering, labeling storage, preparation, and administration of PN admixtures; using double-checks; providing easy access to information about PN) are followed to reduce the risk of errors with PN. Further, the American Society for Parenteral and Enteral Nutrition (A.S.P.E.N.) established the National Advisory Group that developed practice guidelines for "Safe Practices of Parenteral Nutrition Formulations" to assist healthcare organizations in identifying and preventing adverse events associated with PN.

DAILY ORDERING OF PARENTERAL NUTRITION

PN orders are placed daily in CareLink (Computerized Prescriber Order Entry, CPOE). Three different PN order sets are used for pediatric patients based on body weight, and include: PN for less than 10 kg (neonatal), between 10 and 30 kg (pediatric), and more than 30 kg (adolescents). The patient's dosing weight and access route of PN infusion (i.e., central vs. peripheral) must be provided for the PN prescription to proceed in CareLink. PN orders should be renewed daily after evaluating the patient's daily clinical condition, laboratory values, and nutrition requirements. PN orders need to be placed daily in CareLink by 2 PM of the day PN is to be administered. PN orders in CareLink can be placed only for the current day and cannot be placed for future dates.

PN infusion rates should start low and advanced slowly to nutritional goal. This allows metabolic adaptation to dextrose infusion, minimizes the risks of refeeding syndrome, and allows time for adjusting fluids and electrolytes in PN. PN and intravenous lipid emulsions are ordered separately. The volume of intravenous lipid emulsions must also be transcribed into the PN order. The infusion rate for PN and intravenous lipid emulsion are automatically calculated in CareLink to infuse over 24 hours or using a standard pre-built or non-standard cyclic infusion regimen. A summary of daily electrolytes provided in the PN admixture are automatically calculated in CareLink. A PN admixture overfill is automatically added by Pharmacy, with 100 mL overfill added to the adult/adolescent and pediatric PN admixtures, and 50 mL overfill is added to the neonatal PN admixtures.

For adult and adolescent PN (weight over 30 kg) and pediatric PN orders (weight 10 to 30 kg), no more than one liter of central PN or two liters of peripheral PN admixture can be used on the first day of PN. Standard central PN admixtures for adults and adolescents contain dextrose 200 g/L and for pediatrics 150 g/L. Central PN infusion is started at 41 mL/hr on the first day, and increased daily by 20 to 40 mL/hr until the nutritional goal is reached. Fluids and electrolytes are ordered on "per day" basis. Daily multivitamins and trace elements are automatically added per protocol, unless otherwise specified.

For neonatal PN orders (weight less than 10 kg), a total fluid calculator is provided. The patient's total fluid for the day can be entered. The amount of intravenous lipid emulsions must be entered into the total fluid calculator. Additional fluids that the patient is receiving are reported (e.g., fluid from arterial catheters, insulin infusion, vasopressors, enteral nutrition). The total volume of the PN admixture should be ordered to last 24 hours. Amino acids, intravenous lipid emulsions, and electrolytes are ordered on a "per kg" basis. Dextrose can be ordered as dextrose percent in the total PN volume or as a dextrose infusion rate (DIR). The calcium-phosphate compatibility factor is automatically calculated. The default chloride-to-acetate ratio is 1.5-to-1. Daily multivitamins, trace elements, and L-carnitine 5 mg/kg/day are automatically added to the PN of infants who weigh less than 1500 g, unless otherwise specified. Heparin may be added to the PN admixture for patients in the neonatal intensive care unit when indicated (Chapter X).

COMPOUNDING PARENTERAL NUNTRITION ADMIXTURES

Once PN orders are submitted in CareLink, pharmacists evaluate and review the PN formulation. The composition of the PN admixture is determined based on the ability to safely compound the PN ingredients and additives. When indicated, pharmacists recommend adjustments to the PN formulation to ensure physical and chemical compatibility, stability, and sterility of the PN admixture. Thereafter, PN orders are electronically transmitted to an off-site contracted compounding pharmacy. Because PN admixtures are compounded off-site, inpatient pharmacies do not compound PN on-site.

In response to the need of eliminating the risk of patient harm from improperly compounded sterile preparations, the United States Pharmacopeia (USP, the official drug compendium in the United States) first published Chapter <797> titled "Pharmaceutical Compounding: Sterile Preparations" that took effect on January 1, 2004. The Revision Bulletin of USP Chapter <797> was released in late 2007 and the revised version became official on June 1, 2008. The USP Chapter <797> is enforced by the Food and Drug Administration (FDA), and is used by The Joint Commission (TJC) during surveys of hospitals and homecare pharmacies. USP Chapter <797> sets standards, requirements, and procedures to reduce the potential for contamination caused by an unclean environment, pharmacist error, lack of quality assurance, inappropriate compounding, handling and storage, incorrect beyond-use dating, and other factors.

The USP Chapter <797> classifies the risk-level assessment of PN compounding as medium-risk level. Examples of medium-risk level include pooled admixtures compounded using multiple additives and/or small volumes, batch compounded preparations (e.g., syringes) that do not contain bacteriostatic components, complex manipulations and procedures that occur over a prolonged period of time (e.g., PN admixtures), and preparations for use over several days. Medium-risk level product compounding requires the compounding activity in the pharmacy, using appropriate engineering controls (ISO Class 5 hood in an ISO Class 7 clean room). PN compounding by the outsourcing pharmacy meets or exceeds USP Chapter <797> procedures and requirements for PN admixtures used at the University of Michigan Hospitals and Health Centers. PN admixtures are assigned a beyond-use date of 30 hours at controlled room temperature and 9 days under refrigeration.

When compounding a TNA, calcium-phosphate compatibility is based on the lipid-free TNA volume. To avoid lipid coalescence, a minimum of 2% (percentage of the final lipid concentration in solution) intravenous lipid emulsions is necessary in the TNA formulation and compounding. Table 1 describes the differences between 2-in-1 and 3-in-1 PN admixtures.

LATEX ALLERGY: SPECIAL PARENTERAL NUTRITION COMPOUNDING

Latex allergy is caused by antigens contained in latex (processed milky sap of the tree *Hevea brasiliensis*) that can cause an allergic reaction in susceptible individuals. Latex allergy may present as sneezing, rhinoconjunctivitis, hives, wheezing, and respiratory difficulty. Anaphylaxis and serious reactions are more likely to occur with parenteral or mucous membrane contact or by inhalation. High-risk patients for latex allergy include those with myelodysplasia and other neural tube defects, congenital urologic abnormalities, and other conditions necessitating chronic bladder catheterization, or requiring repeated latex exposure as part of a bowel program.

Precautions are taken when compounding and administering PN for latex-sensitive patients. When a latex-free PN admixture is to be compounded, pump tubing is flushed, and the latex-free product is hung with new latex-free tubing and attached to the compounder. For any items that would be added by hand, the one-poke method is used if a latex-free product is not available. Latex-free syringes are used for reconstituting solutions or drawing up additives. For the administration of TNA, a 1.2-micron in-line filter (instead of 0.22-micron filter that is used for 2-in-1 PN admixtures) is used to allow the lipid emulsion particles (about 0.5-micron in diameter) to pass through the filter.

EXPIRATION TIME OF PARENTERAL NUTRITION ADMIXTURES

The expiration time of final PN admixtures is 24 hours from the scheduled administration time. PN admixtures should not be infused into the patient beyond the expiration date and time specified on the PN admixture label, and must be discontinued regardless of the solution volumes remaining after 24 hours from their scheduled administration time.

Table 1. Comparison of Total Nutrient Admixtures and 2-in-1 Parenteral Nutrition Admixtures

Characteristics	Total nutrient admixture (3-in-1)	Parenteral nutrition admixture (2-in-1)
Visual detection of in-solution precipitate (calcium-phosphate)	Cannot be detected, as precipitate is masked by white color of intravenous lipid emulsions	May be detected
In-line filter size and microbial trapping	1.2-micron filter does not trap *Staphylococci* and *E. Coli* microorganisms	0.22-micron filter traps *Staphylococci* and *E. Coli* microorganisms
Y-injection site compatibility	Many medications are incompatible with intravenous lipid emulsions	Several intravenous medications may be co-administered with lipid-free PN admixture, which reduces the need for additional intravenous access
Product wastage	Increased wastage of admixture when admixture is discontinued	Unused unaltered lipid emulsion bottles can be returned to pharmacy for re-use
Number of infusion pumps required	One	Two
Infusion tubing	One tubing per day	One tubing every 96 hours for PN solution without intravenous lipid emulsions. One tubing every 24 hours for intravenous lipid emulsions
Administration time	Usually over 12 to 14 hours in home setting	Mostly over 24 hours in acute care setting
Patient compliance	Simplifies regimen, decreases patient workload, improves patient compliance in home setting	Increased labor demand for patients in home setting

OSMOLARITY OF PARENTERAL NUTRITION ADMIXTURES

Osmolarity is defined as the concentration of osmotically active particles in solution. Osmolarity describes the number of milliosmoles of solute per liter of solvent (mOsm/L). The approximate osmolarity of the adult standard central PN admixture is 1680 mOsm/L. The osmolarity of the adult standard peripheral PN (PPN) admixture is 880 mOsm/L. The osmolarity of the final PN admixture is listed on the PN bag label.

The risk of phlebitis increases with solution osmolarity exceeding 600 mOsm/L, and the maximum tolerated solution osmolarity to infuse via a peripheral vein is 900 mOsm/L. Intravenous lipid emulsions have decreased osmolarity (292 mOsm/L, Liposyn III® 20%) and their co-infusion with the peripheral PN admixture may reduce vein irritation. Contributing factors to phlebitis include high solution osmolarity, extreme pH, prolonged use of the same infusion site, infusion rate, catheter type, and vein properties. PN components that contribute most to the osmolarity of the PN admixture are amino acids and dextrose. Intravenous multivitamins and trace elements have very low osmolarity. The final osmolarity of the PN admixture is the sum of the individual PN components' osmolarity (Table 2).

Table 2. Osmolarities of Parenteral Nutrition Components

PN component	Approximate osmolarity
Amino acids	10 mOsm/g
Dextrose	5 mOsm/g
Intravenous lipid emulsion	0.28 mOsm/mL
Potassium (acetate, chloride, phosphate)	2 mOsm/mEq
Sodium (acetate, chloride, phosphate)	2 mOsm/mEq
Calcium gluconate	1.4 mOsm/mEq
Magnesium sulfate	1 mOsm/mEq

STORAGE OF PARENTERAL NUTRITION DMIXTURES

All PN bags should be stored in a cool place and not exposed to light. Refrigeration of PN admixtures intended for the same day administration is not necessary, as long as the expiration date on the PN label is strictly observed. Although PN admixtures may warm significantly as they pass through the PN administration sets depending on ambient temperature and length of administration sets, refrigerated PN admixtures should be brought close to room temperature for about 2 hours before they are infused into the patient.

INSPECTION OF PARENTERAL NUTRITION ADMIXTURES

Medication administration policies dictate that PN admixtures and labels be inspected and verified by the nurse before PN is infused into the patient:

- PN admixture label should be checked and verified against the original PN order for content, composition, infusion route (central vs. peripheral venous access), infusion volume, and flow rate
- PN admixtures should be inspected for turbidity or precipitates and returned to the pharmacy if not clear

- Intravenous lipid emulsions should be checked for "oiling out" which indicates a break of the emulsion and separation of components, and should not be infused into the patient. Creaming of the lipid emulsion occurs when lipid particles begin to aggregate and migrate to the surface of the emulsion, but can be reversed with mild agitation. If lipid particles continue to aggregate, coalescence may occur, which indicates an irreversible separation of the lipid emulsion. Coalesced intravenous lipid emulsions should not be infused into a patient because they can result in fat emboli
- PN admixtures should not be infused through a peripheral vein if the final dextrose concentration in the PN admixture exceeds 10% for adults and adolescents, and is higher than 12.5% for infants and children
- Intravenous lipid emulsions can be infused via a central or peripheral venous access because they are isotonic solutions
- Intravenous lipid emulsions should be co-infused with peripheral PN admixtures to minimize the risk of phlebitis, unless medically contraindicated
- If the PN admixture is rendered unusable, notify the prescriber

FILTRATION OF PARENTERAL NUTRITION ADMIXTURES

Appropriate in-line filters prevent calcium-phosphate precipitates, lipid aggregates, particulate matter, air, or possible microorganism contaminants from being infused into the patient during PN infusion. Particle sizes of 5 to 20 microns may lodge in the pulmonary capillaries and cause serious or fatal complications (e.g., microvascular pulmonary embolus). Mixed dextrose and amino acid PN admixtures (2-in-1) are filtered through a 0.22-micron pore size bacterial retentive filter. Intravenous lipid emulsion particles are about 0.5 micron and do not pass through a 0.22-micron filter. Intravenous lipid emulsions should be infused via the Y-port below the in-line filter with a 2-in-1 PN admixture. A larger 1.2-micron in-line filter should be used for the 3-in-1 PN admixtures (total nutrient admixtures) to allow the lipid emulsion particles to pass through. The 1.2-micron filter traps *Candida* species, but not *Escherichia coli* or *Staphylococci*.

In-line filters are changed at the same time infusion tubings are changed, which is every 96 hours for the 2-in-1 PN, and every 24 hours for the 3-in-1 lipid-containing PN admixtures. If the filter breaks, cracks, or is clogged, immediately remove the filter and replace it to prevent possible clotting of the venous access.

PARENTERAL NUTRITION ADMIXTURES INFUSION, TUBING, AND CAPS

PN admixtures are delivered to nursing units by 8 PM each day. The standard PN hang time across all patient care units is 9 PM, and the 24-hour PN day starts and finishes at 9 PM the next day.

PN admixtures should be administered by using an infusion pump. Specific guidelines for PN admixture infusion include:

- Two patient identifiers should be used prior to PN administration
- Nurses should record the daily administration of PN on the patient's medication administration record
- Do not attempt to "catch up" on infusion volume or rate
- Notify the prescriber of mechanical or other difficulties that affect the PN flow rate by an amount greater or lesser than 10%
- PN infusion should not be interrupted unless it is medically indicated. Sudden interruption of PN infusion could result in reactive hypoglycemia, with fluid and electrolyte disturbances. If the PN infusion is suddenly interrupted, dextrose 10% in water in adults and adolescents and 12.5% in infants and children should be infused until the next PN bag is available, along with adequate replacement of electrolytes
- Capillary glucose concentrations (i.e., chemsticks or accuchecks) should be monitored 30 minutes after PN is stopped to check for any reactive hypoglycemia. Hypoglycemia should be treated promptly (Chapter XII)
- The intravenous administration set, filter, and extension tubing of PN admixtures without intravenous lipid emulsions must be changed every 96 hours. The intravenous tubing and attached components should be changed every 24 hours for intravenous lipid emulsions
- The tubing used for the infusion of intravenous lipid emulsions must be changed every 24 hours
- Vented tubing is necessary for bottles, but not for plastic bags
- Stopcocks are not to be connected into the PN tubing
- All tubing junctions in Mott Children's Hospital should be taped
- After cleaning of the Y-port below the in-line filter with an alcohol swab, the primed lipid emulsion tubing should be inserted with a locking blunt cannula
- At the time of catheter insertion, a pre-pierced injection port should be used to maintain the system
- All tubing connections and access to the catheter should be made through the pre-pierced injection port using a blunt cannula or a locking blunt cannula
- Pre-pierced caps shall be changed weekly or every 7 days when changing the tubing in the hospital, and whenever blood cannot be flushed from the cap

Discontinuing Parenteral Nutrition Infusion

To discontinue PN, the CareLink PN order should be discontinued to avoid PN wastage and incurred costs. PN should be tapered off slowly before discontinuation, especially in the absence of adequate oral diet or EN that would prevent reactive hypoglycemia. PN should be discontinued before the patient is scheduled for major surgery and can be restarted after surgery.

This avoids fluid, electrolytes, and glucose fluctuations during the surgical procedure. Under the "TPN Management" order option in CareLink, the option for taper PN discontinuation can be used "decrease rate by 50% x 2 hours, then D/C." The other option is "discontinue after current bag" that can be used when the patient has adequate oral or EN intake or an alternative dextrose infusion.

CYCLIC INFUSION OF PARENTERAL NUTRITION ADMIXTURE

PN is infused over 24 hours for most hospitalized patients to minimize glucose, fluid, and electrolyte disturbances. PN administration, via an intermittent infusion or cycle, describes the infusion of the same PN admixture volume over less than 24 hours. A typical PN cycle goal is for PN infusion over 12 hrs. Cyclic PN infusion (e.g., overnight) allows the patient mobility, with freedom from the intravenous poles, infusion pump, and tubing. Cyclic PN infusion also frees the venous access for medication administration. Clinically, cyclic PN reduces the risk for PN-associated cholestasis by avoiding the continuous compulsive nutrient loading to the liver. When patients are expected to receive long-term PN, early PN cycling is recommended.

CareLink automatically calculates standard cyclic infusion rates. The PN cycle is started by "ramping up" the infusion rate over the first 2 hours and "ramping down" the rates over the last 2 hours before PN is disconnected. The remaining volume, minus the volume from the ramping up and down times, is divided by the remaining time of the cycle and infused at a constant rate. Intravenous lipid emulsions do not need to be cycled in a stepwise manner, and are infused at a constant rate over the same PN infusion time. Capillary glucose concentrations are checked at peak infusion rate 4 hours after the initiation of PN cycle to monitor for hyperglycemia, and 30 minutes after PN cycle is completed to monitor for hypoglycemia. Potassium amounts in the PN admixture should be adjusted for the potassium infusion rate not to exceed a maximum of 10 mEq/hr during PN cycling.

A PN cycle for adult and adolescent patents is usually initiated over 18 hours on the first day, then advanced on the second day to 14 to 16 hours, and advanced on the third day to a cycle goal of 10 to 12 hours. Depending on the PN volume, a reasonable approach to cycling PN is to start "ramping up" at 20 to 40 mL/hr on the first hour, and advancing to the second hour at no more than double the first hour rate. PN infusion is "ramped down" over 2 hours in the reverse mode of "ramping up" with the same last hour as the first hour infusion rate. The remaining PN volume minus the volume from the ramping up and down times is divided by the remaining time of the cycle and infused at a constant rate.

A PN cycle for infants and children is usually initiated over 22 hours on the first day, and the cycle is advanced by 2 to 4 hours daily based on tolerance to a cycle goal over 12 hours. Due to their limited glycogen stores, infants may experience fluctuations in serum glucose concentrations when short PN cycles are used.

XVI. PARENTERAL NUTRITION DURING PREGNANCY

INDICATIONS OF PARENTERAL NUTRITION DURING PREGNANCY

Clinical use of parenteral nutrition (PN) during pregnancy is uncommon, especially during the first trimester. Pregnancy itself is not associated with malabsorption or nutrient losses. However, pregnancy is associated with increased energy demands, especially during the second and third trimesters.

Most literature related to PN use in pregnancy is based on case reports. Nonetheless, PN has been successfully and safely used throughout pregnancy until delivery. Common indications of PN during pregnancy are severe hyperemesis gravidarum when oral or enteral nutrition have failed, acute pancreatitis, inflammatory bowel disease, diabetic gastroparesis, bowel obstruction, and anorexia nervosa.

WEIGHT GAIN DURING PREGNANCY

During normal pregnancy, a minimal weight gain of about 0.5 to 2 kg is expected during the first trimester. The Institute of Medicine 2009 revised guidelines for weight gain for singular gestation during pregnancy based on pre-pregnancy body mass index (BMI) are shown
in Table 1.

Table 1. Total and Rate of Weight Gain during Singular Gestation Pregnancy

Pre-pregnancy BMI[a]	Total body weight gain (kg)	Rates of weight gain during 2nd and 3rd trimesters (kg/week)
Underweight (< 18.5)	12.7–18.1	0.45–0.59
Normal weight (18.5–24.9)	11.3–15.9	0.36–0.45
Overweight (> 25–29.9)	6.8–11.3	0.22–0.31
Obese ($\geq$ 30)	5–9.1	0.18–0.27

[a]BMI = body mass index = body weight (kg)/height (m^2).

FLUID AND ELECTROLYTE REQUIREMENTS

Daily maintenance fluid and electrolyte requirements are adjusted as needed based on the patient's hemodynamic parameters, kidney function, and serum electrolyte concentrations (Chapter VI). Acute fluid and electrolyte disturbances, especially occurring with hyperemesis, should be corrected outside the PN admixture. In general, for a total weight gain of 12.5 kg during pregnancy, 7.613 kg is water accumulation.

ENERGY REQUIREMENTS

Pregnancy is an anabolic state and calorie requirements are adjusted to ensure adequate maternal weight gain and fetal tissue accretion. The increase in calorie requirements during pregnancy averages about 150 kcal/day during the first trimester, and 300 kcal/day in the second and third trimesters. One method to estimate energy requirements in pregnant patients is by calculating the basal energy expenditure (BEE) using the Harris-Benedict equation:

BEE= 655 + [9.6 x body weight[a] (kg)] + [1.7 x height (cm)] − [4.7 x age (years)]

[a]Body weight = pre-pregnancy weight.

To account for the factors to support pregnancy (newly synthesized tissues, anabolism, increased basal metabolic rate), total calorie requirements during normal pregnancy can be estimated by adding 150 kcal/day for the first trimester and 300 kcal/day for the second and third trimesters to the BEE. Under hypermetabolic conditions when the hospitalized pregnant patient is on ventilator support, indirect calorimetry should be used for the most accurate estimation of calorie requirements.

A balanced PN regimen provides the following distribution of total daily calories: amino acids 10% to 20%, dextrose 50% to 60% (in the absence of hyperglycemia or diabetes), and intravenous lipid emulsions 20% to 30% (in the absence of hypertriglyceridemia). The optimal dextrose infusion rate should not exceed 4 mg/kg/min.

AMINO ACIDS

Protein or amino acid requirements during pregnancy are approximately 1 g/kg of pre-pregnancy weight plus an additional 10 g/day to support pregnancy. Higher amino acid requirements are needed in pregnant patients under metabolic stress and adjusted based on underlying clinical conditions (see Chapter III).

TRACE ELEMENTS, MINERALS, AND VITAMINS

Data on nutrient requirements in pregnancy are mostly derived from the dietary reference intakes (DRIs), which are based on normal oral nutrient intake (http://www.iom.edu/). However, the application of the DRIs to pregnant patients who have altered metabolic requirements due to disease and stress may be inaccurate. Also, applying the DRIs that are based on oral intake to parenteral intake is also inaccurate as the parenteral route bypasses the gastrointestinal tract and provides 100% bioavailability of nutrients.

Recommended daily parenteral trace element and mineral requirements in normal pregnancy compared to the standard parenteral trace element formulation are shown in Table 2. Vitamin requirements during pregnancy based on the DRIs in comparison with the composition of the adult intravenous multivitamin formulation are shown in Table 3.

Table 2. Daily Parenteral Trace Element and Mineral Intake in Pregnancy Compared with Standard Parenteral Multiple Trace Element (MTE-5[®]) Formulation

	Daily recommended intake in PN during pregnancy[a]	Parenteral Multiple Trace Element (MTE-5[®])-1 mL
Trace elements		
Chromium	10–15 mcg	10 mcg
Copper	0.5–1.5 mg	1 mg
Manganese	0.15–0.8 mg	0.5 mg
Selenium	20–40 mcg	60 mcg
Zinc	2.55–3 mcg	5 mg
Iodine	50 mcg	
Iron	3–6 mg	
Minerals (as electrolytes)		
Calcium	12.5 mEq	
Magnesium	10–15 mEq	
Phosphorus	30–45 mmol	

[a]From: MacBurney M, Wilmore DW. Parenteral nutrition in pregnancy. In: Rombeau JL, Caldwell MD, eds. Parenteral Nutrition. Philadelphia: W.B. Saunders Company;1986:696-715.

MONITORING PARAMETERS

Maternal weight gain and fetal growth should be regularly monitored. Accurate interpretation of laboratory data should consider the normal physiologic changes during pregnancy. For instance, serum albumin concentrations decrease during pregnancy independent of the nutritional status. Further, there are limitations to the sensitivity and specificity of visceral proteins as markers of nutritional status during pregnancy and under metabolic stress (Chapter VII).

Serum iron, ferritin, hemoglobin, hematocrit, and total iron binding capacity (TIBC) are used to monitor iron status. However, serum ferritin concentrations can be increased in response to oxidative stress, inflammation, infection, or liver disease regardless of iron status. During pregnancy, there is also a decrease in serum zinc, calcium, magnesium, and phosphorus concentrations and an increase in serum copper, possibly related to tissue redistribution.

Serum glucose concentrations should be maintained within acceptable range to avoid the complications of hyperglycemia or hypoglycemia (Chapter XII).

Maternal hyperglycemia during pregnancy, even with serum glucose concentrations below those diagnostic of diabetes, can be associated with increased risks of adverse pregnancy outcomes (e.g., increased birthweight and cord-blood serum C-peptide levels). There is also possible correlation between hyperglycemia and risk for premature delivery, shoulder dystocia or birth injury, need for intensive neonatal care, hyperbilirubinemia, and preeclampsia. If hyperglycemia occurs, dextrose calories in PN should be reduced to about 50% of total daily calories and the dextrose infusion rate kept between 2 and 4 mg/kg/min. If these measures alone fail to restore normal serum glucose concentrations, treatment with insulin is recommended. Because insulin requirements during pregnancy differ and change throughout gestation, close monitoring of blood glucose concentrations with adjustments to the insulin dose are necessary.

Lipids are essential for fetal growth and neurologic development and should be regularly provided during pregnancy. Because serum triglyceride concentrations increase in the second and third trimesters, judicious administration of intravenous lipid emulsions with close monitoring of serum triglyceride concentrations is recommended.

Table 3. Vitamin Requirements during Pregnancy Based on Dietary Reference Intakes Compared with Standard Adult Intravenous Multivitamin Formulation

Vitamin	Dietary Reference Intakes (DRIs)[a]	Parenteral MVI Infuvite® Adult-10 mL
Fat-soluble vitamins		
Vitamin A	(as retinol equivalent)	3300 IU (1000 mcg)
≤ 18 y.o.	750 mcg	
19–30 y.o.	770 mcg	
31–50 y.o.	770 mcg	
Vitamin D	5 mcg	200 IU (5 mcg)
Vitamin E	15 mg α-tocopherol	10 IU (10 mg)
Vitamin K		150 mcg
≤ 18 y.o.	75 mcg	
19–30 y.o.	90 mcg	
31–50 y.o.	90 mcg	
Water-soluble vitamins		
Thiamine (B1)	1.4 mg	6 mg
Riboflavin (B2)	1.4 mg	3.6 mg
Niacin	18 mg	40 mg
Pantothenic acid	6 mg	15 mg
Pyridoxine (B6)	1.9 mg	6 mg
Cyanocobalamin (B12)	2.6 mcg	5 mcg
Biotin	30 mcg	60 mcg
Folic acid	600 mcg	600 mcg
Ascorbic acid (C)		200 mg
≤ 18 y.o.	80 mg	
19–30 y.o.	85 mg	
31–50 y.o.	85 mg	

MVI = multivitamins.

[a]From: Food and Nutrition Board, Institute of Medicine, National Academy of Sciences. Dietary Reference Intakes: Recommended Intakes for Individuals, 2001.

XVII. HOME PARENTERAL AND ENTERAL NUTRITION

Home parenteral nutrition (HPN) and home enteral nutrition (HEN) are available for patients requiring long-term nutrition support therapy. Successful home nutrition support therapy requires a strong commitment by the patient and one other close person (e.g., caregiver, family member, friend) who will be available for assistance and support. Individuals must demonstrate the necessary skills for handling HPN or HEN, which include principles of sterile technique, catheter care management, simple compounding and administration skills, and ability to identify therapy-related complications.

Patient education and training should begin early to ensure a safe and timely patient discharge. Because the training process may cause anxiety and overwhelm patients and caregivers, patients to be discharged on HPN or HEN should be referred as soon as possible to the Discharge Planner who covers respective medical or surgical services. The Discharge Planner will verify insurance coverage, identify home infusion providers, and arrange visiting nurse coverage.

HPN and HEN patients are offered the services of HomeMed, the University of Michigan's home infusion program. HomeMed clinicians are available for on-site education, training, and monitoring. They provide interdisciplinary follow-up care, in coordination with the patient's physician, following patient discharge. HomeMed maintains a 24-hour on-call system (phone 800-862-2731) for its home therapy patients.

CANDIDATES FOR HOME NUTRITION SUPPORT THERAPY

Home Parenteral Nutrition

Insurance usually covers HPN-related expenses when patients have severe pathology of the alimentary tract that prohibits the absorption of sufficient nutrients to maintain weight, growth, and strength. Patients must have a condition involving the small intestine and/or its exocrine glands that significantly impairs the absorption of nutrients, or a disease of the stomach and/or intestines, such as motility disorders, that impair the ability of nutrients to be transported through the gastrointestinal tract. In most cases, failed enteral nutrition (EN) is a necessity for approval of HPN insurance coverage. The patient's medical record and discharge summary should show evidence of EN failure. Also, objective evidence should support the underlying diagnosis that necessitates HPN. Additional testing and documentation may be required for patients with certain insurance providers as their primary insurance (e.g., testing for gastrointestinal motility or other bowel studies, documentation of therapeutic interventions, fecal fat measurements, imaging series).

Home Enteral Nutrition

Insurance usually covers HEN-related expenses when patients have nonfunctional segments of the gastrointestinal tract that do not permit food to reach the small intestine, or when a disease of the small intestine impairs food digestion and absorption (e.g., dysphagia, bowel obstruction, gastroparesis). Some insurance providers require a trial of gravity EN (for gastric feeding) before an enteral feeding pump becomes a covered benefit. Documentation of limited gastrointestinal function is also required in the patient medical record. In the case of Medicare, the patient must also have "nothing by mouth" (NPO) and requires full nutrition support via tube feeding for at least 90 days.

INITIATION OF PARENTERAL AND ENTERAL NUTRITION AT HOME

Some patients may qualify for initiation of HPN or HEN at home rather than being admitted to the hospital. Patients must be clinically stable, have proper indication for EN or parenteral nutrition (PN), be evaluated in the home, and have access to visiting nurse services to provide home training on the safe administration of therapy. Patients considered as high risk for nutrition support initiation in the home setting include infants; intravenous drug abusers; patients with major organ dysfunction, poorly controlled diabetes; and those with or at risk for fluid, electrolyte, acid-base imbalances, or refeeding syndrome, who require close and frequent monitoring that cannot be successfully done at home.

PARENTERAL NUTRITION: TRANSITION FROM HOSPITAL TO HOME

HPN is commonly infused over a "cycle" to allow time off the infusion during the day and improve patient's mobility (Chapter XV). It is advised that PN cycling is initiated while the patient is in the hospital to ensure tolerance and address any signs and symptoms of hypoglycemia, hyperglycemia, or fluid and electrolytes imbalances.

A complete set of laboratory parameters should be obtained at least one day prior to patient discharge. Laboratory parameters include a comprehensive metabolic panel (sodium, potassium, chloride, carbon dioxide, blood urea nitrogen, creatinine, glucose, calcium, albumin, protein, liver transaminases, alkaline phosphatase, bilirubin), phosphorus, magnesium, triglycerides, complete blood count, and platelets. Laboratory parameters that are monitored at home usually include weekly comprehensive panel, serum magnesium and phosphorus concentrations. The frequency of laboratory monitoring is decreased to every other week or monthly once the patient is stable on PN. Other specific blood testing (e.g., trace elements, vitamins, carnitine) are obtained according to the patient's specific clinical and disease states.

If a patient receiving HPN is readmitted to the hospital, communication should be made between the prescriber and home-care provider to ensure the appropriate in-hospital PN formulation is ordered.

ENTERAL NUTRITION: TRANSITION FROM HOSPITAL TO HOME

Patients to be discharged on HEN may require adjustments to their hospital EN regimen to allow time off the tube feeding at home. In general, adult patients who are receiving EN into the stomach, via a gastrostomy, Percutaneous Endoscopic Gastrostomy (PEG), or nasogastric tube, should be changed to gravity feeding if tolerated prior to discharge. Gravity feeding is much easier to learn. If a patient requires a pump for enteral feeding, a cyclic EN schedule is usually indicated for home. Most patients prefer overnight enteral feeding. Hospitalized patients are usually initiated on continuous EN and can tolerate rate increases of 10 to 25 mL/hr every 8 to 12 hours. Once the goal of EN volume is reached, a nocturnal schedule can be gradually initiated by decreasing the number of hours of feeding while increasing the feeding rate. If EN is still being administered over 24 hours on the day of discharge, a schedule can be given to the patient to continue the cycle procedure at home. This is accomplished by increasing the administration rate by 10 mL/hr every 1 to 4 days until the overnight EN schedule is reached. If any signs or symptoms of intolerance develop (e.g., diarrhea, cramping, nausea, bloating), the feeding rate should be decreased back to the previously tolerated rate and cycling can be reattempted again in the next few days.

Most pediatric patients with new gastrostomy tubes are placed on a pump for EN rather than gravity feeding. One exception is in infants with a nasogastric tube who are unable to meet the majority of their nutrition requirements by bottle. In this case, the remainder of the nutrition formula that is not taken by mouth is administered by gravity. If a pediatric patient is discharged with an infusion pump, EN is generally administered over 12 hours. If the patient is still on a 24-hour feeding schedule at discharge, the caregiver may begin increasing the feeding rate at home as tolerated by 5 to 10 mL/hr every 1 to 4 days. Because some pediatric patients are unable to tolerate all their large volume EN requirements over 12 hours, additional 2 or 3 bolus feedings are required during the day.

VISITING NURSE SERVICES

The Discharge Planner arranges for a visiting nurse to assist and observe the patient or caregiver's administration technique for HPN or HEN at home. For HPN patients, the visiting nurse is usually also available at home the following day following hospital discharge to help with disconnecting the PN infusion. The patient or caregiver and visiting nurse will determine the frequency of future visits. A signed Continuing Physicians Care Order (CPC) is required to begin visiting nurse services at home.

XVIII. VENOUS ACCESS DEVICES

Central parenteral nutrition (PN) admixtures are hyperosmolar solutions that should only be infused after a satisfactory X-ray confirmation of the tip position of the venous access device (VAD). To avoid mechanical and septic complications, the PN VAD/lumen and administration tubing should only be used for the infusion of the PN admixture, and should not be used for central venous pressure (CVP) readings, or to administer blood products, "piggyback" medications, blood drawing, or fluids. The policy and procedures for VAD flushing, blood drawing, and dressing changes should Refer to the following internal web link for VAD care policies: be followed. http://www.med.umich.edu/i/nursing/policies/ivAccessPolicy0308.pdf

TEMPORARY PERCUTANEOUS VENOUS ACCESS DEVICES

Central VADs are available with single, double, and triple lumens. The number of lumens selected should be based on the patient's clinical condition, and extra lumens that will not be used should be avoided. VAD insertion should be done in a well-controlled environment using strict aseptic techniques.

Antiseptic/Antibiotic Impregnated Central Venous Access Devices

Clinical studies have demonstrated a decrease in VAD-related bloodstream infection with the use of antiseptic/antibiotic impregnated central catheters. At the University of Michigan Hospitals and Health Centers, VADs impregnated with rifampin and minocycline are used in pediatric patient care areas, and VADs impregnated with chlorhexidine and silver sulfadiazine are used for adults. Prior to VAD insertion, patient allergies to these antiseptics/antibiotics should be ruled out. VADs without antiseptics/antibiotics are available as an alternative.

Dressings

- The VAD insertion site shall be evaluated for erythema, inflammation and/or exudate, pain, or tenderness by either visual or tactile inspection every 24 hours and with every dressing change
- Gauze and tape dressings shall be changed every 72 hours or whenever the dressing is wet, loose, or soiled, if the patient complains of pain at the insertion site or if the dressing is removed for any other reason
- Highly permeable transparent dressings shall be changed at least every 7 days or whenever the dressing becomes wet, loose, soiled, or when inspection of the site is necessary
- A customized PICC/Central Line dressing change kit, using gauze or a transparent membrane dressing, is available from Material Services

- If there is a potential for a dressing to become wet, a highly permeable transparent dressing should be used
- If there is bleeding at the insertion site or the patient is diaphoretic, a gauze and tape dressing should be used
- Ointments are not necessary. However, if an ointment is used, it shall be an iodophor type. Apply the ointment after cleansing the insertion site
- The sterility of the VAD cutaneous junction and an occlusive dressing at all times are the cornerstones for VAD longevity. The following directions are for the application of dressings:
    1. Open the sterile PICC/Central Line dressing change kit that contains all the necessary items needed to change the dressing
    2. Put on sterile gloves
    3. Cleanse the area with a 2% CHG in 70% alcohol swabstick (i.e., Chloraprep®) using a back and forth motion with friction for 30 seconds. When cleansing a multilumen VAD, the area from the VAD insertion site to approximately two inches along the VAD should be considered sterile
    4. For gauze and tape dressing:
        a. Cover the insertion site with a folded 4x4 gauze
        b. Place the second folded 4x4 gauze to cover the hub of the VAD and first part of the extension tubing for a single lumen catheter or two inches of the exposed multilumen VAD
        c. Apply skin-prep around the 4x4 gauze; let air dry until smooth and shiny
        d. Apply the tape down the center of the dressing and then pinch the tape around the extension tubing for a single lumen VAD or around the VAD itself for a multilumen VAD to achieve total occlusiveness. Then apply tape on both sides of the first piece of tape
        e. Bring a loop of extension tubing up to the dressing and tape
        f. Write the time, date, and your initials on the dressing
    5. For transparent dressing:
        a. Apply skin-prep approximately one-half inch around the VAD. Let air dry until smooth and shiny
        b. Remove the backing from the dressing
        c. Apply the dressing over the VAD so that the VAD exit site is in the middle of the dressing. Pinch the dressing around the VAD itself to achieve total occlusion
        d. Bring a loop of extension tubing next to the transparent dressing and tape

Catheter Care

- Luer lock extension tubing is mandatory on all central VADs

- Luer lock extension tubing that is connected to the central VAD underneath the dressing should be changed only when the dressing is changed (i.e., every 96 hours)
- The middle lumen of a triple-lumen VAD, and the proximal lumen of a double-lumen VAD, should be designated the PN lumen and should be treated as such for the duration of insertion. The infusion lumen of a pulmonary artery VAD should be utilized for the infusion of the PN admixture
- PN admixtures may be infused through a VAD/lumen that was used for other purposes prior to PN. Once the PN is discontinued, the VAD/lumen may be used for other treatment purposes
- If a lumen of a triple- or double-lumen VAD is no longer needed, it may be maintained with a heparin lock. The unused VAD lumen should be flushed every 24 hours using heparinized saline (10 units/mL) 5 mL in adults and 1 to 3 mL in pediatric patients
- When two lumens of a triple-lumen VAD are no longer needed, it should be replaced with a single-lumen VAD
- Never attempt to push a VAD back into the patient if the VAD has become displaced
- Sutures that are loose or have come out should be replaced by the physician
- A VAD that has become displaced should be anchored with steri-strips or another suture to prevent further VAD movement. The physician should be notified if it is suspected that a VAD has become displaced
- If a VAD is placed in an area of hair growth, the area may be clipped when necessary and scrubbed with a 2% CHG in 70% alcohol swabstick. It is not recommended to use a razor as it may lead to nicks and abrasions resulting in microbial colonization
- The junction of the VAD hub and extension tubing on a single-lumen VAD is considered sterile; therefore, this area is included under the dressing. Microbial contaminants at this junction can migrate down the VAD and enter the bloodstream
- When there is a crack in the lumen hub or exudate at the VAD exit site, the physician should be notified immediately to remove the VAD
- A chest X-ray is mandatory following the replacement of a VAD by the use of a guidewire
- Only nurses with demonstrated competency may remove a VAD

PERIPHERALLY INSERTED CENTRAL CATHETERS

General

A peripherally inserted central catheter (PICC) should be used for PN therapy that is anticipated for greater than 7 days. PICCs are placed by specially trained registered nurses on the Vascular Access Service (VAS) or by Angiography if veins are not accessible for bedside placement. PICC placement requires a physician order via CareLink (Computerized Prescriber

Order Entry, CPOE) specifying the type of VAD required. The VAS nurse will then determine vein accessibility. A signed informed consent is necessary prior to VAD placement. A chest X-ray is required following VAD insertion to confirm that the PICC tip position is in the superior vena cava (SVC). The PICC should not be used until confirmation has been obtained. PICCs can be kept in place indefinitely, barring post-insertion complications. PICCs are removed by the VAS nurse following a written physician order.

Dressings

- PICC dressings are changed by the VAS nurse every 7 days, or when the VAD dressing becomes loose or wet, or for any other emerging reasons
- A transparent membrane dressing is required at all times to cover the PICC insertion site
- A customized PICC/Central Line dressing change kit, using gauze or a transparent membrane dressing, is available from Materiel Services

Catheter Care

- Blood sampling through the PICC should be avoided whenever possible. If a blood draw is necessary, use only a 4.0 French (18-Gauge) single-lumen catheter or the 18-Gauge side of the 5.0 French bi-lumen catheter. Draw with gentle and steady pressure. After sampling is completed in an adult, flush with 10 mL of normal saline followed by 5 mL of heparinized saline (10 units/mL) using a 10 mL syringe. In pediatrics, after blood sampling, flush with 2 mL of normal saline followed by 2 mL of heparinized saline (10 units/mL) using a 10 mL syringe
- Always use a 10 mL syringe when flushing to avoid VAD rupture
- Flush the PICC following intermittent medication administration with 3 mL of heparinized saline (10 units/mL) using a 10 mL syringe in adults, and with 2 mL of heparinized saline in pediatrics
- Flush the PICC once daily when not in use
- If resistance is encountered when flushing, the physician should be notified immediately, as it may be necessary to use a thrombolytic agent to avoid total VAD occlusion
- A continuous infusion of normal saline at 1 to 3 mL/hr must be used for PICCs of 1.9 French (24-Gauge) or less, to maintain VAD potency

MIDLINE VENOUS ACCESS DEVICES

General

Midline VADs are peripheral venous catheters made of highly biocompatible material, and can remain in place for up to 8 weeks. Midline VADs may have a maximum total length of 7 inches. Correct Midline VAD placement is approximately 1 inch below or 2 inches above the antecubital space. The placement decision for midline VADs must be based on the type of IV intravenous therapy to be infused. Patients who may be candidates to Midline VADs include those who require up to 4 weeks of intravenous infusion via a peripheral vein, less than 2 weeks of therapy with poor peripheral venous access, and those requiring few days of infusion of irritant medications (e.g., potassium chloride) or high osmolarity solutions (e.g., peripheral PN admixtures). Physician order in CareLink is needed for placement of a midline VAD.

Dressings

- Dressings on midline VADs are changed by the VAS nurse every 96 hours using a transparent dressing, or when the VAD dressing becomes loose or wet, or for any other emerging reasons.

Catheter Care

- Peripheral PN admixtures of a final dextrose concentration not exceeding 10% in adult patients may be infused through the midline VAD
- When the midline VAD is not in use, it should be flushed with 5 mL (adults) or 2 mL (pediatrics) of heparinized saline (10 units/mL) twice daily
- Immediately following the midline VAD insertion, the patient must keep their arm straight. An arm board is placed and the arm is wrapped with warm compresses for the first 30 to 40 minutes following insertion
- Post-infusion phlebitis occasionally occurs with midline VADs and is treated with warm moist soaks applied to the arm for 30 minutes every 3 to 4 hours for the first 24 hours
- Always use a 10 mL syringe for midline VAD flushing
- Blood sampling is not recommended through the midline VAD
- Blood pressure cuffs and tourniquets should not be placed on the arm in which the midline VAD has been placed

TUNNELED VENOUS ACCESS DEVICES

General

Tunneled VADs (e.g., Broviac®, Hickman®) may be used immediately after insertion, once their proper placement is confirmed by a chest X-ray. The use of the tunneled VAD for purposes other than the infusion of the PN admixture should be avoided whenever possible. A customized PICC/Central Line dressing change kit using gauze or transparent membrane can be used.

Dressings

- Gauze and tape dressings (i.e., Medipore®, Tegaderm with Pad®) should be changed every 72 hours, or whenever the dressing becomes wet or loose, or needs to be changed for any other reason
- Semi-permeable, transparent dressings may be changed every 7 days. Transparent dressings should be changed if the dressing becomes loose, or needs to be changed for any other reason

Catheter Care

- For adult patients, irrigation of the tunneled VAD with 5 mL of a heparinized saline (10 units/mL) should be done daily, after blood has been drawn or administered, and after fluid or medication infusion. For neonates, irrigation is done with 1 to 3 mL of heparinized saline (10 units/mL)
- Padded hemostats or a catheter clamp that are specifically designed for the tunneled VAD should be kept at the patient bedside. If resistance is encountered when the tunneled VAD is irrigated, the physician should be notified immediately, as it may be necessary to use thrombolytic agents in order to prevent total VAD occlusion

CHARTING AND DOCUMENTATION

- Insertion of a central VAD, its location, and any complications should be documented in the patient's medical record
- Drainage or redness at the VAD insertion site, skin breakdown, or VAD irregularities should be documented
- PN infusion should be charted on the patient's medication administration record. The nurse name, PN admixture number, and the time and date of PN administration should be recorded
- Administration of a daily heparin flush solution to maintain the patency of unused, multilumen ports should be recorded on the medication administration record. Include the name of the medication, dose, and the frequency of administration

NURSING POLICIES

- Luer lock extension tubing must be attached to all central VADs
- Only nurses with special training may remove central VADs
- When indicated, nurses may aspirate air or a clot from a central VAD, or gently irrigate a central VAD with normal saline using a 10 mL syringe, using aseptic techniques
- Do not attempt to remove a kink from a central VAD because its manipulation may lead to VAD dislodgment

XIX. TECHNICAL COMPLICATIONS ASSOCIATED WITH CENTRAL VENOUS ACCESS DEVICES

COMPLICATIONS ASSOCIATED WITH INSERTING CENTRAL VENOUS ACCESS DEVICES

Physicians who are experienced in the techniques of subclavian and internal jugular venipuncture can insert a venous access device (VAD) to be used for PN infusion. VAD insertion for PN administration is never an emergency and should only be performed under planned circumstances, with sufficient assistance available and following strict aseptic techniques. Possible complications associated with VAD insertion are shown in Table 1.

Table 1. Possible Complications Associated with VAD Insertion

• Pneumothorax	• Thromboembolism
• Subclavian artery puncture	• Thoracic duct laceration
• Carotid artery injury	• Air embolism
• Hemothorax	• VAD embolism
• Hydromediastinum	• VAD malposition
• Cardiac perforation and tamponade	• Subclavian hematoma
• Brachial plexus injury	• Horner's Syndrome
• Innominate or subclavian vein laceration	• Phrenic nerve injury

Pneumothorax is the most common complication (1% to 2% of attempted catheterizations) associated with subclavian venipuncture. Pneumothorax may be asymptomatic and resolves spontaneously, or the patient may require tube thoracostomy. Instructing patients to hold their breath on deep expiration or temporarily stopping positive pressure mechanical ventilation reduces the incidence of pneumothorax. A chest film is mandatory after every catheterization or replacement of a VAD over a guidewire in order to alert for possible VAD placement-associated complications and to confirm the VAD position before using it.

Subclavian artery puncture is the second most frequent VAD placement-associated complication. It can be minimized by maintaining the angle of the VAD entry close to the horizontal plane. If arterial blood is returned on insertion of the VAD trocar needle, the needle should be withdrawn and direct pressure applied for a minimum of five minutes.

Carotid artery puncture is the most common complication of percutaneous internal jugular vein catheterization. If it is judged that the patient is at low risk for complications, applying firm pressure directly to the puncture site may suffice. If this complication goes unrecognized, the resulting hematoma may enlarge rapidly if the patient is coagulopathic that could lead to tracheal compression, airway obstruction, respiratory compromise, and pseudoaneurysm.

Air embolism is a potentially fatal complication of percutaneous catheterization of the subclavian and internal jugular veins. To minimize the occurrence of air embolism, the patient should be placed in a Trendelenburg position during the removal of the syringe from the needle trocar and passage of the VAD into the vein. Alternatively, the transition should be made rapidly during deep expiration or with mechanical ventilation temporarily interrupted. Air embolism can also occur during routine VAD changes. If a patient is inadvertently disconnected from the VAD or the introduction of air during attempted subclavian or internal jugular vein VAD insertion is suspected, immediate management should consist of clamping off the VAD and placing the patient on the left side down in the Trendelenburg position. If the VAD is in place, an attempt should be made to aspirate the air. Fresh sterile tubing should be connected to the VAD hub when the patient's clinical status permits. If the tubing becomes disconnected proximal (on the bottle side) to the filter, the filter itself will act as an air lock and prevents the patient from siphoning the air into the vascular system.

COMPLICATIONS ASSOCIATED WITH USING CENTRAL VENOUS ACCESS DEVICES

Occlusions

VAD patency is defined by the ability to infuse through the VAD and to withdraw blood from the VAD. Causes, signs, and symptoms of central VAD occlusions are shown in Table 2.

When a VAD becomes occluded, a thorough stepwise assessment should be followed in attempt to identify the types and causes of the occlusion before the VAD can be further used. First, check for mechanical causes such as unopened clamps, sutures, occluded filters, and kinked tubing. Second, check for blood return or by flushing the VAD. Third, ask the patient to raise the ipsilateral arm and shrug their shoulders forward in order to check if the occlusion is cleared by postural changes. Fourth, question the history of the VAD by determining if blood has recently been drawn, or if a medication or blood was infused through the VAD. Fifth, assess the patient for the presence of edema, pain, redness, or dilated vessels around the VAD site.

Table 2. Causes and Signs and Symptoms Associated with Venous Access Device Occlusions

Cause	Signs and symptoms
Intraluminal clotting	Complete occlusion
Intraluminal precipitate	Complete occlusion temporarily related to medication administration
Fibrin sleeve	Infusion with ease, inability to aspirate blood
Pinch-off syndrome	Complete occlusion related to postural changes
VAD malposition	Pain with infusion, swelling, resistance to infusion, inability to aspirate blood
Venous thrombosis	Edema: neck, jaw, and shoulder pain; paresthesia; dilated peripheral vessels
External compression	Complete occlusion related to clamps, sutures, occluded needles

Intraluminal Clotting

Intraluminal thrombus may be due to insufficient VAD flushing, lack of positive pressure when flushing, infusion pump malfunction, blood draws, blood transfusion, and changes in patient intrathoracic pressure. The treatment of an intraluminal VAD clot is to instill the VAD with a thrombolytic agent. It is important that the thrombolytic agent comes into close contact with the thrombus. At the University of Michigan, the recommended thrombolytic of choice for VAD occlusion is urokinase 5,000 units/mL. As an alternative when urokinase is unavailable, Alteplase (t-PA) 1 mg/mL is used. Alteplase 1 mg/mL syringes are good for 6 months at -20 degrees Celsius (-4 degrees Fahrenheit). Alteplase (Cathflo Activase®) 2.5 mg is restricted for hemodialysis catheter clearance only, or may be used for medical procedures other than catheter clearance requiring a low alteplase dose.

Thrombolytic agents should be instilled into an occluded VAD using the negative pressure technique as described below:

1. Gather supplies and establish a clean working environment
2. Apply gloves
3. Keeping the arm below the level of the heart, place sterile 4x4 gauze under the hub of the catheter. Clamp the VAD. Hold the VAD hub with an alcohol pad. Remove the extension set or injection cap from the VAD. Using sterile technique, attach a three-way stopcock to the VAD hub. Make sure the stopcock is in the off position
4. Swab one port of the stopcock with an alcohol pad and attach an empty 10 mL syringe
5. Swab the other port on the stopcock with an alcohol pad and attach a 10 mL syringe containing one dose of the thrombolytic agent. (Note: using two syringes allows the contents of the VAD to be aspirated without the risk of medication incompatibility or contamination)

6. Turn the stopcock off to the thrombolytic syringe and open to the empty 10 mL syringe. Gently aspirate until the plunger is at the 8 to 10 mL mark to create a vacuum
7. Turn the stopcock off to the aspirated syringe and on to the thrombolytic solution syringe. (Note: when this is done, the medication will be automatically drawn into the VAD).
8. Turn the stopcock to the off position, allowing the thrombolytic to remain in the VAD for 30 to 120 minutes
9. Label the VAD with a piece of tape that indicates: "Urokinase (or alteplase) instilled-do not use"
10. Attempt aspiration by opening the stopcock and checking for a blood return every 30 to 120 minutes. Repeat steps 6 through 8 again, if necessary
11. If the VAD patency does not return after 120 minutes, a second dose of thrombolytic may be repeated
12. When VAD patency is restored, aspirate 3 to 4 mL of blood to remove all the thrombolytic and residual clot
13. Remove the stopcock and attach the pre-flushed sterile extension set
14. Following established procedure, flush the VAD with 5 to 10 mL of normal saline and then flush with the appropriate amount of heparin flush or connect to the intravenous infusion
15. Remove the label which indicated that a thrombolytic was instilled
16. Document medication administration and outcome, including any adverse reactions
17. If the VAD declot is unsuccessful, notify the physician for further instructions and possible VAD replacement

Intraluminal Precipitates

Medication incompatibilities, calcium salts, phosphates, antibiotics, intravenous lipid emulsions, and heparin can cause VAD occlusions. There is a higher incidence of intraluminal precipitates caused by coalescence and enlargement of lipid particles with total nutrient admixtures.

Hydrochloric acid 0.1N at 0.2 to 1 mL can be used to treat VAD occlusions caused by calcium-phosphate precipitates. Hydrochloric acid lowers the pH within the VAD lumen and enhances precipitate solubility. Hydrochloric acid has also shown benefits in treating VAD occlusions due to precipitates caused by medications like amikacin, piperacillin, vancomycin, and heparin.

Sodium bicarbonate 8.4% for parenteral use has been used at 1 mEq/mL to restore the patency of occluded VADs with precipitates caused by ticarcillin/clavulanate potassium, oxacillin, and phenytoin.

VAD occlusions caused by intravenous lipid emulsion deposits can be successfully treated by using ethanol (ethyl alcohol) 70% at 3 to 5 mL instilled into the VAD lumen for 1 to 2 hours.

The negative pressure technique should also be used for the instillation of these medications. When a precipitate is suspected, a review of the PN formulation and intravenous medication administration and incompatibilities (Appendix K) is necessary to help determine the cause and avoid future complications.

Occlusions of Unknown Etiology

If the cause of occlusion remains unclear, the first treatment option is to use a thrombolytic. If there is uncertainty as to whether the precipitation is basic or acidic in nature, hydrochloric acid is suggested as the initial treatment.

Extraluminal Thrombus

Fibrin sheaths may form at the end of the VAD tip, making it difficult to draw blood from the VAD. Fibrin sheath may grow over the tip of the VAD causing a fibrin tail (sleeve). If necessary, the diagnosis can be made by injecting dye into the VAD under fluoroscopy.

Treatment usually consists of instilling a thrombolytic inside the VAD. Intraluminal VAD volumes vary (Table 3), but most do not exceed 1 mL. Intraluminal VAD volumes can be estimated as follows:

Intraluminal VAD volume = catheter length (cm) x intraluminal volume (mL/cm)

A thrombolytic (e.g., urokinase or alteplase) volume of 0.8 to 2 mL is instilled using a 10 mL syringe and clamped for 30 minutes (or up to 2 hours) to ascertain that enough thrombolytic reaches the thrombus. This may be repeated a second time if the first attempt fails to declot the VAD. When declotting a peripherally inserted catheter (PICC), the negative pressure technique described above should be used. If the VAD patency cannot be restored following the second thrombolytic dose, the physician should be notified for further treatment options. If necessary, a recent chest x-ray with the current VAD in place can be examined to determine the exact length of the VAD, because the VAD is frequently cut to patient size.

Table 3. Intraluminal Volumes for Venous Access Devices

Venous access device	Intraluminal volume (mL/cm)
Hickman	0.020
Adult Broviac	0.008
Pediatric Broviac	0.004
Baby Broviac	0.002

Pinch-Off Syndrome

Pinch-off syndrome occurs at the narrow triangular area where the axillary vein becomes the subcalavian vein. Pinch-off syndrome does not occur with

PICCs. It occurs during postural changes and is caused by the VAD compression by the clavicle and first rib. Changing the patient positioning by raising the arm usually relieves the VAD obstruction. The diagnosis of pinch-off syndrome is made by either obtaining a chest X-ray that shows a luminal narrowing, or by injecting dye directly into the VAD under fluoroscopy. If pinch-off syndrome is confirmed, the VAD should be removed because of the high risk of breaking and causing VAD fragmentation that may lead to an embolus. The VAD is usually replaced lateral to the midclavicular line.

Malposition and Migration of the Venous Access Device

VAD malposition or migration may occur at any time during VAD longevity. This may be caused by coughing, sneezing, or improper VAD securement. This is especially concerning with unsutured PICCs. It is important that the external length of PICCs and midline VADs be measured following placement, and re-measured if the VAD tip location is not confirmed. Signs and symptoms of VAD malposition or migration include pain during infusion or flushing; sluggish infusion flow rates; frequent infusion pump occlusion alarms; inability to aspirate blood; increased external VAD length; local pain or swelling of the opposite extremity; neurological changes; dyspnea; and VAD migration of more than 4 inches out of the arm from the original insertion length. If any of these signs and symptoms occurs, a chest X-ray should be taken to check for VAD tip location. If the VAD tip is not in the lower half of the SVC above the junction of the SVC and right atrium, attempts should not be made to advance the VAD into the vein or the VAD needs to be removed. The central PN admixture should be stopped and replaced with a peripheral PN admixture with a lower osmolarity, if PN therapy is to continue.

Venous Thrombosis

Thrombi on the vessel wall may adhere to the VAD, which may progress to cause venous thrombosis. Signs and symptoms of venous thrombosis include pain or burning in the neck, chest, or shoulders; swelling of the neck, face, or arm or at the VAD exit site; discomfort in the shoulder or neck; numbing or tingling in the cannulated extremity; development of superficial collateral veins on the chest; periorbital edema; tachycardia; and shortness of breath. The treatment of the VAD-related venous thrombus depends on the severity of the symptoms and the patient clinical status. Consideration should be made if the patient will require future VAD placement and the availability of venous access. The central VAD should be removed if the patient no longer requires central venous access.

Early Stage Mechanical Phlebitis

Early stage mechanical phlebitis can occur anytime within 7 days of antecubital PICC placement. If recognized and treated early, mechanical phlebitis usually resolves within 72 hours. If symptoms worsen, the PICC should be removed. Signs and symptoms that may occur at the PICC insertion site include pain or tenderness, erythema, swelling, and palpable venous cord. The treatment of mechanical phlebitis consists of rest and elevation of the affected extremity, applying low-degree moist heat from a continuous controlled source, and avoidance of excessive physical exertion of the cannulated extremity.

Air Embolus

Air embolism occurs if large amount of air enters into the bloodstream as an immediate bolus. This occurs if there is a break in the intravenous apparatus above the level of the heart, or if the patient takes a deep breath, coughs, sneezes, or laughs while in an upright position. To decrease the risk of air embolus, it is mandatory that all connections on central VADs are leur lock. Patients are instructed to hold their breath when an exchange of tubing is taking place. The risk of air embolus occurring with PICCs is less as VADs are placed below the level of the heart, although the risk of air embolus cannot be completely excluded. Lethal amounts of air emboli in adults have been reported to be between 300 to 500 mL, but may be as little as 100 mL. Signs and symptoms of air embolism include tachycardia, dyspnea, hypoxia, confusion, hypotension, chest pain, nausea, unexplained unconsciousness, and possible death. If any of these complications occur, immediately stop the entry of air, instruct the patient to lie on the left side with feet elevated, activate emergency medical services, and attempt to remove the air by aspirating it with a 10 mL syringe.

Fracture of the Venous Access Device and Embolus Risk

The most frequent cause of VAD fracture is excessive force used during VAD flushing. Other causes may include suturing around the VAD, using clamps and scissors around the VAD during dressing changes, or VAD break during its removal. To prevent VAD fracture, only 10 mL syringes should be used for flushing. A note should be made in the patient medical record describing the length of PICCs, midlines, and tunneled VADs. Following VAD removal, the VAD length should be measured to be certain that the entire length of the VAD has been removed. Signs and symptoms of VAD fracture include leaking, visible rupture, or VAD-related embolus. If the external portion of the VAD is leaking, the VAD should immediately be clamped above the leak. Tunneled VADs can be repaired by using an 18- or 20-Gauge angiocath on a temporary basis, or can be permanently repaired using the appropriate repair kit. PICCs need to be replaced whenever a leak occurs. If a VAD-related embolus occurs or is suspected, immediate medical attention is required. A chest X-ray should be taken. Any VAD fragments can be removed under fluoroscopy in Angiography. If the VAD length is too short or it has entered the pulmonary vasculature, a thoracotomy in the operating room may be necessary.

XX. APPENDIXES

A. Micronutrient Deficiencies, Toxicities, Markers, and Adult Oral Supplementation

B. Adult Enteral Nutrition Formulas

C. Oral Electrolyte Supplements

D. Intravenous Electrolyte Supplements

E. Mineral and Vitamin Oral Supplements

F. Oral Dosage Forms That Should not be Crushed

G. Food-Drug Interactions

H. Parenteral Amino Acid Bulk Solutions

I. Intravenous Replacement Fluids

J. Electrolyte Content of Body Fluids

K. Y-Injection Site Medication Compatibility with Parenteral Nutrition Admixtures

L. Recommended Dietary Allowances for Energy Requirements in Pediatrics

M. Pediatric Enteral Nutrition Formulas

APPENDIX A

MICRONUTRIENT DEFICIENCIES, TOXICITIES, MARKERS, AND ADULT ORAL SUPPLEMENTATION

Nutrient	Signs and symptoms of deficiency	Signs and symptoms of toxicity	Laboratory tests[a]	Oral adult daily dose[b]
Vitamin B1 (Thiamine)	Beriberi: damage to nervous and cardiovascular systems, mental confusion, muscle weakness, calf myalgias, loss of deep tendon reflexes, acidosis, congestive heart failure	None reported with oral thiamine Rare reports of parenteral thiamine causing anaphylactic shock	Erythrocyte transketolase activity	5–30 mg (up to 300 mg in severe deficiency)
Vitamin B2	Angular stomatitis, cheilosis, atrophy of lingual papillae, glossitis, magenta tongue	Photohemolysis in premature infants from moderate excess	Erythrocyte glutathione reductase activity	5–25 mg
Vitamin B6	Personality changes, irritability, depression, filiform hypertrophy of lingual papillae, aphthous stomatitis, nasolabial seborrhea, forehead rash	Sensory neuropathy, degeneration of dorsal root ganglia	Erythrocyte glutamic-oxaloacetic transaminase activity	10–25 mg (50–300 mg for drug-induced peripheral neuritis; 200–600 mg to treat B6-responsive sideroblastic anemia)
Vitamin B12	Macrocytic megaloblastic anemia, neurologic symptoms from demyelination of spinal cord and brain, sore tongue, weakness, neuropsychiatric manifestations	None reported	Serum vitamin B12, CBC, MCV, 24-hour urine methylmalonic acid (MMA)	0.1–1 mg (2 mg sublingual)

MICRONUTRIENT DEFICIENCIES, TOXICITIES, MARKERS, AND ADULT ORAL SUPPLEMENTATION

Nutrient	Signs and symptoms of deficiency	Signs and symptoms of toxicity	Laboratory tests[a]	Oral adult daily dose[b]
Folic acid	Macrocytic megaloblastic anemia, atrophy of lingual papillae, glossitis	None reported	Serum, red blood cell folate[c]	0.5–1 mg
Niacin	Pellagra: dermatitis, diarrhea, dementia, depression, fatigue	Low cholesterol, vascular dilation, arrhythmias, gastrointestinal symptoms	Blood niacin	10–20 mg (up to 500 mg to prevent or treat pellagra)
Vitamin A	Dry, scaling skin, follicular hyperkeratosis, dry conjunctiva, hypogeusesthesia	Hepatomegaly, musculoskeletal pain, malaise, tenderness, fever, ophthalmoplegia, scleral icterus, sunburn-like eruption, dry scaling skin, cirrhotic-like syndrome, pseudotumor cerebri	Serum retinol, retinyl esters, carotene Dark adaptation test	5,000–50,000 units
Vitamin C	Scurvy, gingivitis, petechial hemorrhage, ecchymoses, erythema	Nausea, vomiting, diarrhea, scorbutic changes	Serum vitamin C Leucocyte vitamin C	100–500 mg
Vitamin D	Rickets, bow legs, osteomalacia, low serum calcium and phosphorus, elevated alkaline phosphatase, hyperparathyroidism	Hypercalcemia, hypercalciuria, anorexia, nausea, vomiting, demineralization of bone	Serum 25-hydroxy-vitamin D	5,000–50,000 units of ergocalciferol (supplement with oral calcium, if needed)
Vitamin E	Hemolysis, neurologic abnormalities	Gastrointestinal upset, fatigue, weakness, dizziness, headache, blurred vision, coagulopathy	Serum vitamin E Serum vitamin E-to-total lipids ratio[d]	60 mg[e] (up to 300 mg for severe vitamin E deficiency)

MICRONUTRIENT DEFICIENCIES, TOXICITIES, MARKERS, AND ADULT ORAL SUPPLEMENTATION

Nutrient	Signs and symptoms of deficiency	Signs and symptoms of toxicity	Laboratory tests[a]	Oral adult daily dose[b]
Vitamin K	Elevated prothrombin time	None reported with oral dosing	Prothrombin time	2.5–25 mg[f]
Iron	Pallor, fatigue, microcytic hypochromic anemia, tachycardia	Hepatomegaly, diabetes, hemo-chromatosis	CBC, MCV, hemo-globin, hematocrit, TIBC, serum iron	2–3 mg/kg elemental iron in 2 to 3 divided doses[g]
Iodine	Goiter, hypothyroidism	Hyper-thyroidism	Urine iodine Thyroid screening and tests	400 mcg (di-iodotyrosine for endemic goiter) 150–300 mcg (potassium iodide)
Zinc	Acrodermatitis enteropathica, growth retardation, hypogonadism, hair loss, immune deficiencies, night blindness, diarrhea, hypogeusesthesia, delayed wound healing	Copper deficiency, microcytic anemia, impaired immunity	Serum zinc	2.5–15 mg elemental zinc[h]
Copper	Hypochromic anemia not responsive to iron, neutropenia, osteopenia, steely hair	Vomiting, hepatic necrosis, ataxia, cirrhosis	Serum copper and cerulo-plasmin	2–3 mg elemental copper (cupric sulfate)

MICRONUTRIENT DEFICIENCIES, TOXICITIES, MARKERS, AND ADULT ORAL SUPPLEMENTATION

Nutrient	Signs and symptoms of deficiency	Signs and symptoms of toxicity	Laboratory tests[a]	Oral adult daily dose[b]
Manganese	Scaly dermatitis, retarded hair and nail growth, hypercalcemia, increased prothrombin time not responsive to vitamin K, hyperphosphatemia, elevated alkaline phosphatase	Hallucinations, extensive neural damage, nephritis, pancreatitis	Serum manganese Red blood cell manganese	2–5 mg elemental manganese
Chromium	Neuropathy, high free-fatty acids, glucose intolerance not responsive to insulin	None reported from dietary excess, industrial exposure	Serum chromium Glucose tolerance test	200 mcg
Selenium	Cardiomyopathy, muscle pain, weakness, macrocytosis, skin and hair depigmentation, glucose intolerance	Hair loss, nail changes, peripheral neuropathy, garlic breath, fatigue	Serum selenium Red blood cell glutathione peroxidase activity	70 mcg[i]

[a]May not be routinely available in most clinical laboratories.

[b]Estimated from available literature. Patients with malabsorption may likely require parenteral supplementation of these vitamins and minerals.

[c]Low serum folate indicates only negative folate balance and not folate deficiency. Red blood cell folate reflects folate status at the time red blood cells were produced. Red blood cell folate is a more reliable indicator of tissue folate deficiency and is not affected by daily variations, such as due to diet.

[d]Alpha tocopherol is the predominant form of vitamin E in the body. A vitamin E-to-total lipids ratio of less than 0.6 to 0.8 mg of vitamin E per 1 g of total lipids is suggestive of vitamin E deficiency. Total lipid concentrations are calculated from the serum cholesterol and triglyceride concentrations. Serum vitamin E concentrations are expressed in mg/L, while serum cholesterol and triglyceride concentrations are in mg/dL.

[e]Tocopherol equivalents: 1 mg dl-alpha tocopheryl acetate = 1 IU; 1 mg dl-alpha tocopherol = 1.1 IU; 1 mg d-alpha tocopheryl acetate = 1.36 IU; 1 mg d-alpha tocopherol = 1.49 IU; 1 mg d-alpha tocopheryl acid succinate = 1.21 IU; 1 mg dl-alpha tocopheryl acid succinate = 0.89 IU.

[f]In patients who underwent gastrectomy or terminal ileum resection, injectable vitamin K is required to correct vitamin K deficiency and maintain normal vitamin K stores.

[g]Elemental iron content of iron salts: ferrous fumarate = 33%; ferrous sulfate anhydrous = 30%; ferrous sulfate = 20%; ferrous gluconate = 11.6%.
[h]Elemental zinc content of zinc salts: zinc oxide = 80%; zinc chloride = 48%; zinc acetate = 30%; zinc sulfate = 23%; zinc gluconate 14.3%.
[i]Intravenous selenium formulation (40 mcg/mL) can be given orally.

APPENDIX B

ADULT ENTERAL NUTRITION FORMULAS AVAILABLE ON FORMULARY

GENERIC NAME	NON-STRESSED FORMULA	STANDARD FORMULA	FIBER FORMULA	HIGH-PROTEIN FORMULA	1.5 CAL/mL FORMULA	2 CAL/mL FORMULA	RENAL LOW-PROTEIN FORMULA	RENAL FORMULA	RENAL LOW-PROTEIN NO-ELECTROLYTES FORMULA	METABOLIC-STRESS FORMULA	CHEMICALLY DEFINED	ENCEPHALOPATHY FORMULA
TRADE NAME	Nutren 1.0	Osmolite 1.2	Fibersource HN	Promote	Osmolite 1.5	Nutren 2.0	Suplena with Carb Steady	Nepro with Carb Steady	Renalcal	Crucial	Peptamen Unflavored/ Vanilla	Nutrihep Unflavored
Description	Isotonic tube-feeding formula	Isotonic tube-feeding formula	Fiber-containing tube-feeding formula	Stress/Trauma tube-feeding or oral supplement	High-calorie tube feeding	High-calorie, tube-feeding or oral supplement	Renal disease tube-feeding or oral supplement	Renal disease tube-feeding or oral supplement	Renal disease tube-feeding or oral supplement	Metabolic-stress tube feeding with immunomodulatory ingredients	Elemental tube feeding	Hepatic disease branched chain amino acids
kcal/mL	1.0	1.2	1.2	1.0	1.5	2.0	1.8	1.8	2.0	1.5	1.0	1.5
Protein Source gm/L	40 Calcium and potassium caseinate	55.5 Sodium and calcium caseinate	53 Soy protein isolate Soy protein concentrate	62.5 Sodium and calcium caseinate	62.7 Sodium and calcium caseinate	80 Calcium and potassium caseinate	45 Sodium caseinate Milk protein isolate	81 Calcium, magnesium, and sodium caseinate Milk protein isolate	34.4 Whey protein concentrate Amino-acid blend	94 Enzymatically hydrolyzed casein	40 Enzymatically hydrolyzed whey	40 Crystalline-L amino acids Whey protein concentrate
Fat Source gm/L	38 Canola oil Corn oil MCT Soy lecithin	39.3 High-oleic safflower oil Canola oil MCT Soy lecithin	39 Canola oil MCT	26 Safflower oil Canola oil MCT	49.1 High-oleic safflower oil Canola oil Soy lecithin MCT Corn oil	104 Canola oil Corn oil Soy lecithin	96 High-oleic safflower oil Canola oil Soy lecithin	96 High-oleic safflower oil Canola oil Soy lecithin	82.4 MCT Canola oil Corn oil Soy lecithin	67.6 MCT Soybean oil Fish oil Soy lecithin	39 MCT Sunflower oil Soy lecithin	21.2 MCT Canola oil
Carbohydrate Source gm/L	127 Corn syrup solids	157.5 Corn maltodextrin	160 Corn syrup	130 Corn maltodextrin Sucrose	203.6 Corn maltodextrin	196 Corn syrup	205 Corn maltodextrin Sucrose	167 Corn syrup solids Sucrose	290.4 Maltrodextrin	134 Maltrodextrin	127 Maltodextrin	290 Maltodextrin Modified cornstarch
Sodium* mg (mEq)/L	876 (38)	1340 (58.3)	1200 (52)	1000 (43.5)	1400 (60.9)	1300 (56.5)	785 (34)	1060 (46.1)	0	1168 (50.8)	560 (24.3)	160 (7)
Potassium* mg (mEq)/L	1248 (32)	1810 (46.4)	2000 (51)	1980 (50.8)	1800 (46)	1920 (49.2)	1120 (28.6)	1060 (27.2)	0	1872 (48)	1500 (37.5)	1320 (33)
Non-Protein Kcal/gm Nitrogen	133:1	110:1	115:1	75:1	125:1	131:1	227:1	115:1	300:1	57:1	131:1	209:1
Volume to meet 100% RDA, mL	1500	1000	1165	1000	1000	750	948	948	1000 (for 9 water-soluble vitamins)	1000	1500	1000
mOsm/kg Water	315	360	490	340	525	745	600	585	600	490	270 Unflavored 380 Flavored	790
Free Water mL/L	848	820	814	839	762	703	735	725	700	772	850	760
Phosphorus* mg/L	668	1200	1000	1200	1000	1340	700	700	0	1000	700	1000
Comments	Kosher Gluten-free Lactose-free Low-residue Unflavored	Kosher Gluten-free Lactose-free Low-residue Unflavored	Kosher Lactose-free — may be suitable for Gluten-free diet 10g/L fiber	Lactose-free Gluten-free Low-residue Kosher Vanilla flavor	Gluten-free Lactose-free Low-residue Kosher Unflavored	Lactose-free Gluten-free Low-residue Kosher	Gluten-free Lactose-free Low-residue Kosher 16g fiber/L	Lactose-free Gluten-free Low-residue Kosher 16g fiber/L	Lactose-free Gluten-free Low-residue Kosher	Lactose-free Gluten-free Low-residue	Lactose-free Gluten-free Low-residue Not palatable	Lactose-free Gluten-free Low-residue Kosher Not palatable

APPENDIX B (continued)

ADULT ENTERAL NUTRITION FORMULAS AVAILABLE ON FORMULARY

ORAL SUPPLEMENTS

TRADE NAME	Nestle Carnation Instant Breakfast Lactose-Free	Nestle Carnation Instant Breakfast VHC	Nestle Carnation Instant Breakfast No Sugar Added	Nestle Carnation Instant Breakfast Packet	Peptamen 1.5	ReGen HP/HC	Resource Breeze Juice Drink	Mighty Shake	Scandi Shake
Container/Serving Size	250 mL/can	250 mL/can	20 gm packet (270 mL)	36 gm packet (270 mL)	250 mL/can	6 oz carton (180 mL)	8 oz box (237 mL)	4 oz carton (120 mL)	3 oz packet mixed w/ 8 oz whole milk
Description	Canned oral food supplement	Canned oral food supplement Vanilla flavored	Reduced calorie and carbohydrate oral food supplement Van or Choc flavored	Low-fat oral food supplement Van/Choc/Straw flavored	Canned oral food supplement Vanilla flavored	Renal oral supplement Van/Straw flavored	Clear liquid oral supplement Orange or Wild Berry flavored	Oral supplement Van/Choc/Straw flavored	High-calorie oral supplement Choc/Van flavored
kcal/serving	250	560	140 w/skim milk	250 w/low-fat milk	375	375/345	250	200	600 w/whole milk
Protein Source gm/serving	8.75 Calcium Caseinate	22.5 Calcium Caseinate Potassium Caseinate Isolated soy protein	13	13	16.9 Enzymotically hydrolyzed whey protein	12/14	9 Whey protein isolate	6	14
Fat Source gm/serving	9.2 Canola oil Corn oil Soy lecithin	30.6 Canola oil Corn oil Soy lecithin	0.5	5	14 MCT oil Soy oil Soy lecithin	17/16	0	6	29
Carbohydrate Source gm/serving	33.1 Corn syrup solids Sugar	49.2 Corn syrup solids Sugar	23 Maltodextrin	38 Maltodextrin Sugar	47 Maltodextrin Corn starch	47/35	54 Sucrose Corn syrup Corn syrup solids	29	65
Sodium* mg (mEq)/serving	219 (9.5)	290 (12.6)	180 (7.8)	220 (9.6)	255 (11)	180 (7.8)/ 188 (8.2)	80 (3.5)	60 (2.6)	230 (10)
Potassium* mg (mEq)/serving	312 (8)	440 (11.3)	706 (18.1)	617 (15.8)	465 (12)	23 (0.6)/ 30 (0.8)	20 (0.5)	150 (3.8)	970 (24.9)
Volume to meet 100% RDA, mL	2100	750	1080 (4 svg)	1080 (4 svg)	1000	-	-	-	-
mOsm/kg Water	490	950	-	-	550	-	750	-	-
Free Water mL/serving	213	168	-	-	193	-	195	-	-
Phosphorus* mg/serving	125	306	497	482	250	68/90	160	100	515
Comments	Kosher Lactose-free Gluten-free Cholesterol-free Low-residue	Kosher Lactose-free Gluten-free Low-residue	Kosher Gluten-free Calorie-restricted Low-residue	Contains Lactose Oral Supplement	Lactose-free Elemental oral or tube-feeding	Kosher Low-lactose Low-sodium	Kosher Lactose-free Low-residue	Kosher Gluten-free	Kosher Gluten-free
Oral Supplement Charge to Patient	Yes	Yes	Yes	Yes	Yes	Yes	Yes	No	Yes

MODULARS

TRADE NAME	Resource Beneprotein	Polycose	Resource Benefiber
Container/Serving Size	7 gm packet	1T = 6gm	4gm packet
Description	Protein modular	Glucose polymer module	Fiber modular
Kcal/mL	25 kcal per scoop or packet	23 kcal per Tbsp	16 kcal Tbsp or packet
Protein Source gm/scoop or packet	6 Whey protein isolate	0	0
Carbohydrate Source gm/scoop or packet	0	5.6	4 (3 gm fiber) High-fructose corn syrup Sugar
Sodium* mg per scoop or packet	10	7.8	15
Potassium* mg per scoop or packet	35	0.6	15
Phosphorus* mg per scoop or packet	15	0.9	-
Comments	Fat-free	Kosher Gluten-free Lactose-free	Fat-free
Oral Supplement Charge to Patient	Yes	Yes	Dispensed from Pharmacy

* Values calculated for Vanilla flavor; other flavors may vary in regards to sodium, potassium, and phosphorus.

APPENDIX C

ORAL ELECTROLYTE SUPPLEMENTS AVAILABLE ON FORMULARY

Oral electrolyte supplements	Dosage forms and composition
Bicarbonate salts	Sodium bicarbonate tablets 650 mg (sodium 7.7 mEq; bicarbonate 7.7 mEq) Sodium bicarbonate oral liquid 1 mEq/mL
Calcium salts	Calcium carbonate suspension 250 mg/mL (elemental calcium 100 mg) Calcium carbonate tablets 1250 mg (elemental calcium 500 mg) Calcium carbonate tablets 1500 mg (elemental calcium 600 mg) Calcium carbonate chewable tablets 500 mg (elemental calcium 200 mg) Calcium acetate oral gelcap 667 mg Calcium chloride oral liquid 20 mg/mL Calcium gluconate oral liquid 100 mg/mL Calcium citrate/Vitamin D3 315 mg/200 units Calcium phosphate tribasic (TCP) 150 mg powder, 39% elemental calcium 150 mg TCP mixed in 100 mL of feeding formula provides 60 mg calcium and 28 mg phosphorus
Magnesium salts	Magnesium oxide tablets 400 mg (elemental magnesium 241.3 mg = ~ 20 mEq) Magnesium gluconate 1000 mg/5 mL (elemental magnesium 54 mg) Magnesium sulfate oral solution 500 mg/mL
Phosphate salts	Sodium phosphate oral solution 0.05 mmol/mL, 0.12 mmol/mL, 3 mmol/mL Potassium phosphate 3 mmol/mL Neutra-phos® oral packets (sodium phosphate/potassium phosphate) (250 mg = elemental phosphorus 8 mmol, potassium 7.1 mEq, sodium 7.1 mEq)
Potassium salts	Potassium chloride extended release tablets 10 mEq, 20 mEq Potassium chloride oral powder packet for reconstitution 20 mEq Potassium acetate oral solution 2 mEq/mL
Sodium salts	Sodium chloride/potassium chloride tablets 450 mg/30 mg

APPENDIX D

INTRAVENOUS ELECTROLYTE SUPPLEMENTS USED IN THE MAKING OF PARENTERAL NUTRITION ADMIXTURES

Intravenous electrolyte salt	Pharmacy bulk solution concentration
Potassium acetate	2 mEq/mL
Potassium chloride	2 mEq/mL
Potassium phosphate[a]	3 mmol/mL
Sodium acetate	2 mEq/mL
Sodium chloride	4 mEq/mL
Sodium phosphate[b]	3 mmol/mL
Magnesium sulfate[c]	4 mEq/mL
Calcium gluconate[d]	0.45 mEq/mL

[a]1 mmol potassium phosphate yields 1.47 mEq of elemental potassium.
[b]1 mmol sodium phosphate yields 1.33 mEq of elemental sodium.
[c]1 g magnesium sulfate is equivalent to 8.1 mEq of elemental magnesium.
[d]1 g calcium gluconate is equivalent to 4.56 mEq of elemental calcium.

APPENDIX E

MINERAL AND VITAMIN ORAL SUPPLEMENTS AVAILABLE ON FORMULARY

Single Oral Mineral Supplements

Oral mineral supplement	Oral dosage forms
Copper gluconate	Capsule 2 mg
Fluoride	Sodium Fluoride drops 0.5 mg/mL
Iron salts	Ferrous sulfate solution 75 mg/0.6 mL (drops); 100 mg/5 mL; 300 mg/5 mL Ferrous sulfate tablets 324 mg (elemental iron 65 mg) Ferrous gluconate tablets 300 mg Iron polysaccharide capsule 150 mg Iron polysaccharide elixir 20 mg/mL
Selenium	Tablet 50 mcg; Oral liquid compounded at desired dose
Zinc salts	Zinc sulfate 220 mg (elemental zinc 50 mg) Zinc sulfate suspension, compounded, 44 mg/mL (elemental zinc 10 mg/mL)

Single Oral Vitamin Supplements

Oral vitamin supplement	Oral dosage forms
Vitamin A, Aquasol A[®]	Capsules 10,000 units; Solution 50,000 units/mL
Ascorbic acid (C)	Solution 90 mg/mL (drops); Tablets 250, 500 mg
Cyanocobalamin (B12)	Tablets 100, 500 mcg
Ergocalciferol (D2 Calciferol)	Capsules 50,000 units (1.25 mg); Solution compounded 1,000 units/mL Solution Drisdol[®] 60 mL: 8,000 units (200 mcg)/mL, 200 units/drop (40 drops/mL)
Cholecalciferol (D3)	Tablets 400 units; Solution drops 400 unit/mL
Folic acid	Tablets 1 mg, scored; Solution 200 mcg/mL
Phytonadione (K1)	Tablets 5 mg, scored; Liquid 2 mg/mL
Pyridoxine (B6)	Tablets 25, 50 mg; Suspension 10 mg/mL
Thiamine (B1)	Tablets 50, 100 mg; Suspension 25 mg/mL

Tocopherols (E)
  Tocopherol acetate, D, L, Alpha Aquasol E[®] **drops**
  Tocopherols concentrate, mixed
  Water-soluble vitamin E, Tocopherols +
  Tocotrienols, Aqua-E[®]
	Solution 50 units/mL (drops)
	Capsules 100, 400 units
	Solution 20 units/mL, 100 IU (d-alpha-Tocopherol) + 156 mg (Tocopherols and Tocotrienols)/5 mL

Refer to the inpatient Pharmacy Formulary website
http://ummcpharmweb.med.umich.edu/formulary/
for complete list of products on Formulary.

APPENDIX F

ORAL DOSAGE FORMS THAT SHOULD NOT BE CRUSHED[1]

Drug product	Dosage form	Reasons/comments[2]
Accutane	Capsule	Mucous membrane irritant
Aciphex	Tablet	Slow release
Actiq	Lozenge	Slow release; lollipop delivery system requires patient to slowly allow dissolution
Actonel	Tablet	Irritant: chewed, crushed, or sucked tablet may cause oropharyngeal irritation
Adalat CC	Tablet	Slow release
Adderall XR	Capsule	Slow release (a)
AeroHist Plus	Tablet	Slow release (h)
Afeditab CR	Tablet	Slow release
Aggrenox	Capsule	Slow release
Alendronate	Tablet	Slow release
Allegra-D	Tablet	Slow release
Allerest Allergy Sinus 12-Hour	Tablet	Slow release
Allfen Jr.	Tablet Capsule	Slow release Slow release (a)
Alpophen	Tablet	Enteric-coated
Alprazolam ER	Tablet	Slow release
Altoprev	Tablet	Slow release
Ambien CR	Tablet	Slow release
Amitiza	Capsule	Slow release
Amrix	Capsule	Slow release
Aplenzin	Tablet	Slow release
Aptivus	Capsule	Taste: oil emulsion with spheres
Aquatab C	Tablet	Slow release (h)
Aquatab D	Tablet	Slow release (h)
Arthrotec	Tablet	Enteric-coated
Asacol	Tablet	Slow release
Ascriptin A/D	Tablet	Enteric-coated
Augmentin XR	Tablet	Slow release (b, h)
Avinza	Capsule	Slow release (a, not to be mixed with pudding)

ORAL DOSAGE FORMS THAT SHOULD NOT BE CRUSHED[1]

Drug product	Dosage form	Reasons/comments[2]
Avodart	Capsule	Drug may cause fetal abnormalities; women who are or may become pregnant should not handle capsules; all women should use caution in handling capsules, especially leaking capsules
Azulfidine EN-tabs	Tablet	Enteric-coated
Cardizem LA	Tablet	Slow release (a)
Bayer Enteric-Coated	Caplet	Enteric-coated
Bayer Low Adult	Tablet	Enteric-coated
Bayer Regular Strength	Caplet	Enteric-coated
Bellahist-D LA	Tablet	Slow release
Biaxin-XL	Tablet	Slow release
Bidhist	Tablet	Slow release
Bidhist-D	Tablet	Slow release
Biltricide	Tablet	Taste (h)
Biohist LA	Tablet	Slow release (h)
Bisac-Evac	Tablet	Enteric-coated (c)
Bisacodyl	Tablet	Enteric-coated (c)
Bisa-Lax	Tablet	Enteric-coated (c)
Boniva	Tablet	Irritant: do not chew or suck, potential for oropharyngeal ulceration
Bromfed PD	Capsule	Slow release
Budeprion SR	Tablet	Slow release
Calan SR	Tablet	Slow release (h)
Carbatrol	Capsule	Slow release (a)
Cardene SR	Capsule	Slow release
Cardizem	Tablet	Although not described as slow release, it has a coating intended to release the drug over a period of about 3 hours
Cardizem CD	Capsule	Slow release (a)
Cardizem LA	Tablet	Slow release (a)
Cardura XL	Tablet	Slow release
Cartia XT	Capsule	Slow release
Ceclor Extended-Release	Tablet	Slow release
Ceftin	Tablet	Taste (b); use suspension for children

ORAL DOSAGE FORMS THAT SHOULD NOT BE CRUSHED[1]

Drug product	Dosage form	Reasons/comments[2]
Cefuroxime	Tablet	Taste (b); use suspension for children
CellCept	Capsule, Tablet	Teratogenic potential (i)
Charcoal Plus	Tablet	Enteric-coated
Chlor-Trimeton 12-Hour	Tablet	Slow release (b)
Cipro XR	Tablet	Slow release
Claritin-D 12-Hour	Tablet	Slow release
Claritin-D 24-Hour	Tablet	Slow release
Colace	Capsule	Taste (e)
Colestid	Tablet	Slow release
Commit	Lozenge	Integrity compromised by chewing or crushing
Concerta	Tablet	Slow release
Cotazym-S	Capsule	Enteric-coated (a)
Covera-HS	Tablet	Slow release
Creon 5, 10, 20	Capsule	Enteric-coated (a)
Crixivan	Capsule	Taste; capsule may be opened and mixed with fruit puree (e.g., banana)
Cymbalta	Capsule	Slow release (a), may add to apple juice
Cytoxan	Tablet	Drug may be crushed but company recommends using injection
Cytovene	Capsule	Skin irritant
Dallergy	Tablet	Slow release (b, h)
Dallergy-JR	Capsule	Slow release
Deconamine SR	Capsule	Slow release (b)
Depakene	Capsule	Slow release mucous membrane irritant (b)
Depakote	Capsule	Enteric-coated
Detrol LA	Capsule	Slow release
Dilacor XR	Capsule	Slow release
Dilatrate-SR	Capsule	Slow release
Dilt-CD	Capsule	Slow release
Dilt-XR	Capsule	Slow release
Ditropan	Tablet	Slow release
Doxidan	Tablet	Enteric-coated (c)
DriHist SR	Tablet	Slow release (h)
Drisdol	Capsule	Liquid-filled (d)

ORAL DOSAGE FORMS THAT SHOULD NOT BE CRUSHED[1]

Drug product	Dosage form	Reasons/comments[2]
Drixoral Allergy Sinus	Tablet	Slow release
Drixoral Cold/Allergy	Tablet	Slow release
Drixoral Nondrowsy	Tablet	Slow release
Droxia	Capsule	Exposure to the powder may cause serious skin toxicities; healthcare workers should wear gloves to administer
Drysec	Tablet	Slow release (h)
Dulcolax	Tablet	Enteric-coated (c)
DuraHist	Tablet	Slow release (h)
DuraHist D	Tablet	Slow release (h)
Duraphen II DM	Tablet	Slow release (h)
Duraphen Forte	Tablet	Slow release (h)
Duratuss	Tablet	Slow release (h)
Duratuss A	Tablet	Slow release (h)
Duratuss PE	Tablet	Slow release (h)
DynaCirc CR	Tablet	Slow release
Dynex	Tablet	Slow release (h)
Easprin	Tablet	Enteric-coated
EC-Naprosyn	Tablet	Enteric-coated
Ecotrin Adult Low Strength	Tablet	Enteric-coated
Ecotrin Maximum Strength	Tablet	Enteric-coated
Ecotrin Regular Strength	Tablet	Enteric-coated
Ed A-Hist	Tablet	Slow release (b)
E.E.S. 400	Tablet	Enteric-coated (b)
Effer-K	Tablet	Effervescent tablet (f)
Effervescent Potassium	Tablet	Effervescent tablet (f)
Effexor XR	Capsule	Slow release
Efidac/24	Tablet	Slow release
Efidac/24 Pseudoephedrine	Tablet	Slow release
E-Mycin	Tablet	Enteric-coated
Enablex	Tablet	Slow release
Entex LA	Capsule	Slow release (b)
Entex PSE	Capsule	Slow release

ORAL DOSAGE FORMS THAT SHOULD NOT BE CRUSHED[1]

Drug product	Dosage form	Reasons/comments[2]
Entocort EC	Capsule	Enteric-coated (a)
Equetro	Capsule	Slow release (a)
Ergomar	Tablet	Sublingual form (g)
Ery-Tab	Tablet	Enteric-coated
Erythrocin Stearate	Tablet	Enteric-coated
Erythromycin Delayed-Release	Capsule	Enteric-coated pellets (a)
Evista	Tablet	Taste; teraotogenic potential (i)
ExeFen PD	Tablet	Slow release (h)
Extendryl JR	Capsule	Slow release
Extendryl SR	Capsule	Slow release (b)
Feen-a-mint	Tablet	Enteric-coated (c)
Feldene	Capsule	Mucous membrane irritant
Fentora	Tablet	Buccal tablet; swallow whole
Feosol	Tablet	Enteric-coated (b)
Feratab	Tablet	Enteric-coated (b)
Fergon	Tablet	Enteric-coated
Fero-Grad 500 mg	Tablet	Slow release
Ferro-Sequels	Tablet	Slow release
Flagyl ER	Tablet	Slow release
Fleet Laxative	Tablet	Enteric-coated (c)
Flomax	Capsule	Slow release
Focalin XR	Capsule	Slow release (a)
Fosamax	Tablet	Mucous membrane irritant
Gleevec	Tablet	Taste (h); may be dissolved in water or apple juice
Glipizide	Tablet	Slow release
Glucophage XR	Tablet	Slow release
Glucotrol	Tablet	Slow release
Glumetza	Tablet	Slow release
Guaifed	Capsule	Slow release
Guaifed-PD	Capsule	Slow release
Guaifenesin/ Pseudoephedrine	Tablet	Slow release
Guaifenex DM	Tablet	Slow release (h)
Guaifenex GP	Tablet	Slow release
Guaifenex PSE	Tablet	Slow release (h)
GuaiMAX-D	Tablet	Slow release
H 9600 SR	Tablet	Slow release
Halfprin 81	Tablet	Enteric-coated

ORAL DOSAGE FORMS THAT SHOULD NOT BE CRUSHED[1]

Drug product	Dosage form	Reasons/comments[2]
Heartline	Tablet	Enteric-coated
Hista-Vent DA	Tablet	Slow release (h)
Hydrea	Capsule	Exposure to the powder may cause serious skin toxicities; healthcare workers should wear gloves to administer
Imdur	Tablet	Slow release (h)
Inderal LA	Capsule	Slow release
Indocin SR	Capsule	Slow release (a, b)
Innopran XL	Capsule	Slow release
Intelence	Tablet	Tablet should be swallowed whole and not crushed; tablet may be dispersed in water
Invega	Tablet	Slow release
Isochron	Tablet	Slow release
Isoptin SR	Tablet	Slow release (h)
Isordil Sublingual	Tablet	Sublingual form (g)
Isosorbide Dinitrate Sublingual	Tablet	Sublingual form (g)
Isosorbide SR	Tablet	Slow release
Kadian	Capsule	Slow release (a); pellets disruption may cause a potentially fatal overdose of morphine; can give as a sprinkle on apple sauce or via nasogastric tube
Kaletra	Tablet	Film-coated
Kaon CL-10	Tablet	Slow release (b)
Keppra	Tablet	Taste; some extemporaneous formulas are prepared in the pharmacy
Ketek	Tablet	Slow release (b)
Klor-Con	Tablet	Slow release (b)
Klor-Con M	Tablet	Slow release (b, h)
Klotrix	Tablet	Slow release
K-Lyte	Tablet	Effervescent tablet (f)
K-Lyte CL	Tablet	Effervescent tablet (f)
K-Lyte DS	Tablet	Effervescent tablet (f)
K-Tab	Tablet	Slow release (b)
Lescol XL	Tablet	Slow release
Lesvinex Timecaps	Capsule	Slow release

ORAL DOSAGE FORMS THAT SHOULD NOT BE CRUSHED[1]

Drug product	Dosage form	Reasons/comments[2]
Levbid	Tablet	Slow release (h)
Lexxel	Tablet	Slow release
Lialda	Tablet	Slow release
Lipram 4500	Capsule	Enteric-coated (a)
Lipram PN 10, 16, 20	Capsule	Enteric-coated, slow release (a)
Lipram UL 12, 18, 20	Capsule	Enteric-coated, slow release (a)
Liquibid-D 1200	Tablet	Slow release (h)
Liquibid-PD	Tablet	Slow release (h)
Lithobid	Tablet	Slow release
Lodrane 24	Capsule	Slow release
Lodrane 24D	Capsule	Slow release
Lohist 12-Hour	Tablet	Slow release
Luvox CR	Capsule	Slow release
Maxifed DM	Tablet	Slow release (h)
Maxifed DMX	Tablet	Slow release (h)
Maxiphen DM	Tablet	Slow release (h)
Medent DM	Tablet	Slow release
Mestinon Timespan	Tablet	Slow release (b)
Metadate ER	Tablet	Slow release
Metadate CD	Capsule	Slow release (a)
Methylin ER	Tablet	Slow release
Metoprolol ER	Tablet	Slow release
Micro K Extendcaps	Capsule	Slow release (a, b)
Mifortic	Tablet	Slow release
Miraphen PSE	Tablet	Slow release
Modane	Tablet	Enteric-coated (c)
Morphine Sulfate Extended-Release	Tablet	Slow release
Motrin	Tablet	Taste (e)
Moxatab	Tablet	Slow release
MS Contin	Tablet	Slow release (b)
Mucinex	Tablet	Slow release
Mucinex DM	Tablet	Slow release
Muco-Fen-DM	Tablet	Slow release (h)
Naprelan	Tablet	Slow release
Nasatab LA	Tablet	Slow release (h)
Nexium	Capsule	Slow release (a)

ORAL DOSAGE FORMS THAT SHOULD NOT BE CRUSHED[1]

Drug product	Dosage form	Reasons/comments[2]
Niaspan	Tablet	Slow release
Nicotinic Acid	Capsule, Tablet	Slow release (h)
Nifediac CC	Tablet	Slow release
Nifediac XL	Tablet	Slow release
Nifedipine Extended-Release	Tablet	Slow release
NitroQuick	Tablet	Sublingual route (g)
Nitrostat	Tablet	Sublingual route (g)
Norpace CR	Capsule	Slow release form within a special capsule
Ondrox	Tablet	Slow release
Opana ER	Tablet	Slow release; tablet disruption may cause a potentially fatal overdose of oxymorophone
Oracea	Capsule	Slow release
Oramorph SR	Tablet	Slow release (b)
OxyContin	Tablet	Slow release; tablet disruption may cause a potentially fatal overdose of oxycodone
Palcaps (all)	Capsule	Enteric-coated (a)
Pancrease MT	Capsule	Enteric-coated (a)
Pancrecarb MS	Capsule	Enteric-coated (a)
Pancrelipase	Capsule	Enteric-coated (a)
Panocaps	Capsule	Enteric-coated (a)
Panocaps MT	Capsule	Enteric-coated (a)
Paxil CR	Tablet	Slow release
Pentasa	Capsule	Slow release
PhenaVent D	Tablet	Slow release (h)
PhenaVent LA	Capsule	Slow release
Plendil	Tablet	Slow release
Pre-Hist-D	Tablet	Slow release (h)
Prevacid	Capsule	Slow release
Prevacid SoluTab	Tablet	Orally disintegrating; do not swallow; dissolve in water only and dispense via dosing syringe or nasogastric tube
Prevacid Suspension	Suspension	Slow release; contains enteric-coated granules; mix with water only; not for use in nasogastric tubes
Prilosec	Capsule	Slow release
Prilosec OTC	Tablet	Slow release
Pristiq	Tablet	Slow release

ORAL DOSAGE FORMS THAT SHOULD NOT BE CRUSHED[1]

Drug product	Dosage form	Reasons/comments[2]
Procardia XL	Tablet	Slow release
Profen II	Tablet	Slow release (h)
Profen II DM	Tablet	Slow release (h)
Profen Forte	Tablet	Slow release (h)
Profen Forte DM	Tablet	Slow release (h)
Propecia	Tablet	Women who are, or may become pregnant should not handle crushed or broken tablets
Proquin XR	Tablet	Slow release
Proscar	Tablet	Women who are, or may become pregnant should not handle crushed or broken tablets
Protonix	Tablet	Slow release
Prozac Weekly	Tablet	Enteric-coated
Pseudo CM TR	Tablet	Slow release (h)
Pseudovent	Capsule	Slow release (a)
Pseudovent 400	Capsule	Slow release (a)
Pseudovent DM	Tablet	Slow release (h)
Pseudovent-PED	Capsule	Slow release (a)
Pytest	Capsule	Radiopharmaceutical
QDALL	Capsule	Slow release
QDALL AR	Capsule	Slow release
Ralix	Tablet	Slow release (h)
Ranexa	Tablet	Slow release
Razadyne ER	Capsule	Slow release
Renagel	Tablet	Tablets expand in liquid if broken or crushed
Rescon	Tablet	Slow release (h)
Rescon JR	Tablet	Slow release (h)
Rescon MX	Tablet	Slow release (h)
Respa-1st	Tablet	Slow release (h)
Respa-DM	Tablet	Slow release (h)
Respahist	Capsule	Slow release (a)
Respaire 60 SR	Capsule	Slow release
Respaire 120 SR	Capsule	Slow release
Resperdal M-Tab	Tablet	Orally disintegrating; do not chew or break tablet; after dissolving under tongue, tablet may be swallowed
Revlimid	Capsule	Teratogenic potential; healthcare workers should avoid contact with capsule contents/body fluids

ORAL DOSAGE FORMS THAT SHOULD NOT BE CRUSHED[1]

Drug product	Dosage form	Reasons/comments[2]
Ritalin LA	Capsule	Slow release (a)
Ritalin SR	Tablet	Slow release
R-Tanna	Tablet	Slow release
Rythmol SR	Capsule	Slow release
Santura XL	Capsule	Slow release; capsule may be opened and pellets mixed in water or placed on tongue and swallowed; do not crush or chew pellets
Seroquel XR	Tablet	Slow release
Simcor	Tablet	Slow release
Sinemet CR	Tablet	Slow release (h)
SINUvent PE	Tablet	Slow release (h)
Slo-Niacin	Tablet	Slow release (h)
Solodyn	Tablet	Slow release
Somnote	Capsule	Liquid-filled
Sprycel	Tablet	Film-coated; active ingredients are surrounded by a wax matrix to prevent healthcare exposure; women who are, or may become pregnant should not handle crushed or broken tablets
Stahist	Tablet	Slow release
Strattera	Capsule	Capsule content can cause ocular irritation
Sudafed 12-Hour	Capsule	Slow release (b)
Sudafed 24-Hour	Capsule	Slow release (b)
Sular	Tablet	Slow release
Symax Duotab	Tablet	Slow release
Symax SR	Tablet	Slow release
Taztia XT	Capsule	Slow release (a)
Tegretol-XR	Tablet	Slow release
Temodar	Capsule	If capsules are accidentally opened or damaged, rigorous precautions should be taken to avoid inhalation or contact of contents with the skin or mucous membranes (i)
Tessalon Perles	Capsule	Swallow whole; temporary local anesthesia of the oral mucosa and choking could occur
Theo-24	Capsule	Slow release; contains beads that dissolve throughout the gastrointestinal tract
Tiazac	Capsule	Slow release (a)

ORAL DOSAGE FORMS THAT SHOULD NOT BE CRUSHED[1]

Drug product	Dosage form	Reasons/comments[2]
Topamax	Tablet	Taste
	Capsule	Taste (a)
Toprol XL	Tablet	Slow release (h)
Touro CC-LD	Tablet	Slow release (h)
Touro LA-LD	Tablet	Slow release (h)
Tracleer	Tablet	Women who are, or may become pregnant should not handle crushed or broken tablets
Trental	Tablet	Slow release
Tylenol Arthritis	Tablet	Slow release
Ultram ER	Tablet	Slow release; tablet disruption may cause a potentially fatal overdose of tramadol
Uniphyl	Tablet	Slow release
Urocit-K	Tablet	Wax-coated
Uroxatral	Tablet	Slow release
Valcyte	Tablet	Teratogenic and irritant potential (i)
Verapamil SR	Tablet	Slow release (h)
Verelan	Capsule	Slow release (a)
Verelan PM	Capsule	Slow release (a)
Vesicare	Tablet	Enteric-coated
Videx EC	Capsule	Slow release
Voltaren XR	Tablet	Slow release
VoSpire ER	Tablet	Slow release
Wellbutrin SR, XL	Tablet	Slow release
Xanax XR	Tablet	Slow release
Zolinza	Capsule	Irritant; avoid contact with skin or mucous membranes; avoid contact with crushed or broken tablets
ZORprin	Tablet	Slow release
Zyban	Tablet	Slow release
Zyflo CR	Tablet	Slow release

(a) Capsule may be opened and the contents taken without crushing or chewing; soft food such as applesauce or pudding may facilitate administration; contents may generally be administered via nasogastric tube using an appropriate fluid provided entire contents are washed down the tube.

(b) Liquid dosage forms of the product are available; however, dose, frequency of administration, and manufacturers may differ from that of the solid dosage form.

(c) Antacids and/or milk may prematurely dissolve the coating of the tablet.

(d)   Capsule may be opened and the liquid contents removed for administration.

(e)   The taste of this product in a liquid form would likely be unacceptable to the patient; administration via nasogastric tube should be acceptable.

(f)   Effervescent tablets must be dissolved in the amount of diluent recommended by the manufacturer.

(g)   Tablets are made to disintegrate under the tongue.

(h)   Tablet is scored and may be broken in half without affecting release characteristics.

(i)   Skin contact may enhance tumor production; avoid direct contact.

Common Abbreviations for Extended-Release Products

CR	controlled release
CRT	controlled release tablet
LA	long acting
SR	sustained release
TR	time release
TD	time delay
SA	sustained action
XL	extended release
XR	extended release

Adapted with permission from: Mitchell JF.
http://www.ismp.org/Tools/DoNotCrush.pdf (accessed 2009, September 4).

[1]Correspondance regarding this list may be addressed to:
    John Mitchell, PharmD, FASHP
    Email: rxmitchell@wowway.com

[2]Two official USP terms are used to designate special-release medication forms: "extended release" and "delayed release." Others such as "sustained release," controlled release," etc., are commonly used on package labeling. The term "slow release" is being used here to signify all such drugs with a special release mechanism.

For questions related to medication administration, contact the Drug Information Service (phone 734-936-8200) during work hours, or the 24-hour inpatient satellite Pharmacies (Mott Children's Hospital Pharmacy, phone 734-764-8208; Main Hospital 6th floor satellite Pharmacy, phone 734-936-8251).

APPENDIX G

FOOD-DRUG INTERACTIONS

Generic drug name	Drug brand name	Drug use/indication	Food effect on drug	Patient instructions
Amprenavir	Agenerase®	Anti-HIV	High-fat food decreases absorption Contains vitamin E exceeding daily Reference Intakes (DRIs)	Do not take drug with a high-fat meal Do not take vitamin E supplements
Antilipemic agents: Lovastatin Simvastatin	Mevacor® Zocor®	Used to lower high blood cholesterol	Grapefruit juice increases serum drug concentrations, which may increase risk for skeletal muscle toxicity	Do not use grapefruit juice while taking the drug Orange juice may be used
Atazanavir	Reyataz®	Anti-HIV	Food increases absorption	Take drug with food
Atovaquone	Mepron®	Antiprotozoal	Fatty foods increase absorption	Take drug consistently with meals
Bisphosphonates: Alendronate Etidronate Risedronate	Fosamax® Didronel® Actonel®	Inhibit bone resorption Used to treat hypercalcemia, Paget's disease, osteoporosis	Foods, dairy foods, beverages reduce absorption	Take drug at least one hour before the first food or beverage, on an empty stomach with a full glass of water Do not take with food, juice, mineral water, or coffee Avoid concurrent consumption of dairy foods Remain seated upright for 30 minutes after taking the drug
Calcium Channel Blockers: Amlodipine Nifedipine Verapamil Nimodipine	Norvasc® Procardia® Isoptin® Nimotop®	Antihypertensives, Antianginals Antiarrhytmic Used to treat neurological deficit post-subarachnoid hemorrhage	Grapefruit juice increases absorption or Inhibits metabolism	Avoid grapefruit juice while taking this drug Orange juice may be used

FOOD-DRUG INTERACTIONS

Generic drug name	Drug brand name	Drug use/indication	Food effect on drug	Patient instructions
Cyclosporine	Sandimmune® Neoral® Gengraf®	Immunosuppressant	Serum concentrations vary with different foods Grapefruit juice inhibits metabolism	Take drug consistently in relation to meals Mix oral solution consistently with same liquid (e.g. chocolate milk, orange, or apple juice) Do not use grapefruit juice or eat grapefruits while taking this medication
Delavirdine	Rescriptor®	Anti-HIV	Stomach acid enhances absorption	Patients with decreased stomach acid may take drug with acidic juice such as orange or cranberry juice
Didanosine	Videx®	Anti-HIV	Food decreases absorption	Take drug on empty stomach 1 hour before or 2 hours after meals Chew tablets Tablets and powder may be mixed with water Do not take drug with juice or acidic liquids
Efavirenz	Sustiva®	Anti-HIV	High fat food increases absorption leading to increased adverse events	Do not take drug with high-fat meals Take on empty stomach
Furazolidone	Furoxone®	Antibacterial Antiprotozoal	Tyramine-rich foods can cause hypertensive crisis	Avoid tyramine-rich foods such as aged cheeses, red wine, beer, avocados, liver, aged or spoiled foods
Indinavir	Crixivan®	Anti-HIV	Heavy meals decrease absorption	Take drug preferably on empty stomach May take drug with a light meal or snack Take drug 1 hour before or 2 hours after large meals May take drug with water, skim milk, coffee, tea

FOOD-DRUG INTERACTIONS

Generic drug name	Drug brand name	Drug use/indication	Food effect on drug	Patient instructions
Isoniazid	INH®	Antimicrobial Antitubercular	Tyramine-rich foods can cause hypertensive crisis	Avoid tyramine-rich foods such as aged cheeses, red wine, beer, avocados, liver, aged or spoiled foods
Itraconazole	Sporanox®	Antifungal	Grapefruit juice impairs absorption Food enhances the absorption of oral capsules Fasting enhances the absorption of oral solution	Do not use grapefruit juice while taking the drug Oral capsules should be taken with meals Oral suspension should be taken on empty stomach
Linezolid (injection and oral dose forms)	Zyvox®	Antibiotic	Tyramine-rich foods can cause hypertensive crisis	Avoid tyramine-rich foods such as aged cheeses, red wine, beer, avocados, liver, aged or spoiled foods
Monoamine Oxidase Inhibitors (MAOI): Isocarboxazid Phenelzine Tranylcypromine	Marplan® Nardil® Parnate®	Antidepressants	Tyramine- and dopamine-rich foods can cause hypertensive crisis	Avoid tyramine-rich foods such as aged cheeses, red wine, beer, avocados, liver, aged or spoiled foods Avoid dopamine-rich foods such as broad (fava) beans
Nelfinavir	Viracept®	Anti-HIV	Food enhances absorption	Take drug with food
Phenytoin	Dilantin®	Anticonvulsant, used to control seizures	Enteral feedings cause decrease in serum phenytoin concentrations	With tube feedings, hold feeding for 1 hour before and 1 hour after administration of phenytoin
Posaconazole	Noxafil®	Antifungal	High-fat food and liquid nutritional supplement significantly increase absorption	Take drug with fatty meal or Boost Plus®
Procarbazine	Matulane®	Antineoplastic	Tyramine-rich foods can cause hypertensive crisis	Avoid tyramine-rich foods such as aged cheeses, red wine, beer, avocados, liver, aged or spoiled foods

FOOD-DRUG INTERACTIONS

Generic drug name	Drug brand name	Drug use/indication	Food effect on drug	Patient instructions
Ritonavir	Norvir®	Anti-HIV	Food enhances absorption	Take drug with food May mix oral solution with chocolate milk to improve taste
Saquinavir	Invirase® Fortovase®	Anti-HIV	Food enhances absorption	Take drug with food
Sirolimus	Rapamune®	Immunosuppressant	Fatty foods decrease absorption Grapefruit juice inhibits metabolism	Take drug consistently in relation to meals Do not use grapefruit juice or eat grapefruits while taking the drug May take this medication with orange juice Do not use grapefruit juice when mixing the sirolimus solution form
Tacrolimus	Prograf®	Immunosuppressant	Fatty foods decrease absorption Grapefruit juice inhibits metabolism	Take drug consistently in relation to meals Do not use grapefruit juice or eat grapefruits while taking this medication May take this medication with orange juice
Voriconazole	VFEND®	Antifungal	Fatty foods decrease absorption and maximum serum drug concentration	Take tablets and suspension at least one hour before or after a meal
Warfarin	Coumadin®	Anticoagulant	Vitamin K in diet decreases drug effects Food alters absorption	Maintain consistent vitamin K dietary intake Take drug consistently in relation to meals
Zidovudine	Retrovir®	Anti-HIV	Fatty food decreases absorption	Do not take drug with fat meals Take drug on empty stomach 1 hour before or 2 hours after meals

APPENDIX H

PARENTERAL AMINO ACID BULK SOLUTIONS AVAILABLE ON FORMULARY

Solution description	FreAmine III[®] 10%[a] (BBraun)	Aminosyn II[®] 15%[a] (Hospira)	Trophamine[®] 10%[b] (BBraun)
Amino acid concentration	10%	15%	10%
Nitrogen (g/L)	15.3	23	15.5
Protein equivalent (g/L)	95.6	150	97
Essential amino acids (mg/100 mL)			
Isoleucine	690	990	820
Leucine	910	1500	1400
Lysine	730	1575	820
Methionine	530	258	340
Phenylalanine	560	447	480
Threonine	400	600	420
Tryptophan	150	300	200
Valine	660	750	780
Nonessential amino acids (mg/100 mL)			
Alanine	710	1490	540
Arginine[c]	950	1527	1200
Histidine[c,d]	280	450	480
Proline	1120	1083	680
Serine	590	795	380
Taurine[e]			25
Tyrosine[c,d]		405	240
Glycine	1400	750	360
Glutamic acid		1107	500
Aspartic acid		1050	320
Cysteine[d]	< 16		< 16
Electrolytes			
Sodium (mEq/L)	10	58.1	5
Chloride (mEq/L)	< 3		< 3
Acetate (mEq/L)	89	107.6	97
Phosphate (mmol/L)	10		
Osmolarity (mOsm/L)	950	1300	875
pH	6–7	5–6.5	5–6
Antioxidants (per 100 mL)			
Sodium bisulfite	< 100 mg		
Sodium hydrosulfite		20 mg	
Sodium metabisulfite			< 50 mg

[a]Amino acid solutions for patients receiving parenteral nutrition with body weight $\geq$ 10 kg. FreAmine III[®] 10% is the Formulary product of choice for patients who weigh $\geq$ 10 kg. Aminosyn II[®] 15% is restricted to patients who weigh $\geq$ 10 kg with persistent hyperphosphatemia despite restrictions in phosphate intake.
[b]Amino acid solutions for patients receiving parenteral nutrition with body weight < 10 kg.
[c]Conditionally essential or indispensable in patients with kidney failure.
[d]Essential or indispensable in infants.
[e]Conditionally essential or indispensable in infants, particularly very low birthweight infants.

158

APPENDIX I

INTRAVENOUS REPLACEMENT FLUIDS

Composition of Standard Intravenous Replacement Fluids

Intravenous solution	Dextrose (g/L)	Electrolytes (mEq/L)				
		Na	Cl	K	Ca	Lactate[a]
D5W (dextrose 5%)	50					
D10W (dextrose 10%)	100					
D50W (dextrose 50%)	500					
3% NaCl		513	513			
0.9% NaCl (NS)		154	154			
0.45% NaCl (1/2 NS)		77	77			
0.225% NaCl (1/4 NS)		38.5	38.5			
D5W 0.9% NaCl	50	154	154			
D5W 0.45% NaCl	50	77	77			
D5W 0.225% NaCl	50	38.5	38.5			
Lactated Ringer's		130	109	4	3	28

NaCl = sodium chloride; NS = normal saline; Na = sodium; Cl = chloride; K = potassium; Ca = calcium.

[a]Lactate is metabolized in vivo in the liver to bicarbonate in a 1:1 molar ratio.

APPENDIX J

ELECTROLYTE CONTENT OF BODY FLUIDS

Composition of Body Fluids and Secretions[a]

Type	Electrolytes (mEq/L)				
	Na^+	K^+	Cl^-	HCO_3^- [b]	H^+
Gastric	40–100	5–25	90–140		90
Biliary	120–154	5–12	80–110	35–50	
Pancreatic	110–154	5–12	50–120	70–110	
Ileostomy	80–130	5–10	50–60	50–70	
Diarrhea[c]	25–50	35–60	70–115	30–45	
Urine[c]	30–80	30–80	50–100		

Na^+ = sodium ion; K^+ = potassium ion; Cl^- = chloride ion; HCO_3^- = bicarbonate ion; H^+ = hydrogen ion.

[a]Amounts of electrolyte losses vary. Other electrolytes (e.g., magnesium, phosphorus, calcium) may also be lost depending on source and severity.

[b]In case of bicarbonate deficit, acetate can be increased in the parenteral nutrition formulation to correct for bicarbonate losses when correction of the acid-base disorder is not urgent. Acetate is converted in vivo to bicarbonate at a 1:1 molar ratio, and the conversion is rapid but not immediate. Sodium bicarbonate is the mainstay of therapy when rapid correction of acidosis is indicated or the patient is symptomatic.

[c]Significant magnesium losses also occur, especially in severe conditions or with specific medication therapy.

"Y"-INJECTION SITE MEDICATION COMPATIBILITY WITH PARENTERAL NUTRITION ADMIXTURES[a]

Medication	2-in-1 PN	3-in-1 PN (TNA)	Intravenous lipid emulsions[a]
Acetazolamide	I		
Acyclovir	I	I	I
Albumin, Human	C[b]	I	I
Aldesleukin (Interleukin-2)	C		C
Amikacin	C	C/I[c]	[c]
Aminophylline	C	C	C
Amoxicillin sodium	C/I		
Amphotericin B	I		I
Ampicillin	C/I	C/I	I
Ampicillin-sulbactam	C	C	
Argatroban	C		
Ascorbic acid	C		[d]
Atracurium besylate	C		[e]
Aztreonam	C	C	C
Bumetanide	C	C	C
Buprenorphine HCl	C	C	C
Butorphanol tartrate	C	C	C
Carboplatin	C	C	C
Cefamandole	C	C	C
Cefazolin	C[f]	C	C
Cefotaxime	C	C	C
Cefotetan	C	C	C
Cefoxitin	C	C	C
Ceftazidime	C	C	C
Ceftizoxime	C	C	C
Ceftriaxone[g]	C	C	C
Cefuroxime	C	C	C
Chloramphenicol	C		C
Chlorothiazide	I		
Chlorpromazine	C		C
Cimetidine hydrochloride	C	C	C
Ciprofloxacin	I	C	C[e]
Cisplatin	I	C	C
Clindamycin phosphate	C	C	C
Clonazepam	C		
Cloxacillin	C	C/I	[h]
Cyanocobalamin	C		I
Cyclophosphamide	C	C	C

"Y"-INJECTION SITE MEDICATION COMPATIBILITY WITH PARENTERAL NUTRITION ADMIXTURES[a]

Medication	2-in-1 PN	3-in-1 PN (TNA)	Intravenous lipid emulsions[a]
Cyclosporine	C/I	C/I	C
Cytarabine	I	C	C
Dexamethasone	C	C	C
Digoxin	C	C	C
Diphenhydramine	C	C	C
Dobutamine	C	C	C
Dopamine	C	C/I	C/I
Doxorubicin hydrochloride	I	I	I
Doxycycline	C	I	I
Droperidol	C	I	I
Enalaprilat	C	C	C
Epinephrine	C		
Epoetin Alfa	C		
Erythromycin lactobionate	C	C	C
Famotidine	C		C
Fentanyl	C	C	C
Floxacillin	C		
Fluconazole	C	C	C
Fluorouracil	I	I	C/I
Folic acid	C	C	C
Foscarnet	C		
Furosemide	C/I	C	C
Ganciclovir	I	I	I
Gentamicin	C	C	C
Granisetron	C	C	C
Haloperidol	C	I	I
Heparin	C	I[i]	I[i]
Hydrocortisone sodium phosphate/succinate	C	C	C
Hydromorphone	C	C/I	C/I
Hydroxyzine	C	C	C
Idarubicin	C		
Ifosfamide	C	C	C
Imipenem-cilastatin	C	C	C
Immune globulin intravenous	C		
Insulin, regular	C	C	C
Iron dextran	C	I	I
Isoproterenol		C	C

"Y"-INJECTION SITE MEDICATION COMPATIBILITY WITH PARENTERAL NUTRITION ADMIXTURES[a]

Medication	2-in-1 PN	3-in-1 PN (TNA)	Intravenous lipid emulsions[a]
Kanamycin	C	C	C
Leucovorin	C	C	C
Lidocaine hydrochloride	C		C
Lorazepam	C	I	I
Mannitol	C	C	C
Meperidine hydrochloride	C	C	C
Meropenem		C	C
Mesna	C	C	C
Methotrexate	I	C	C
Methyldopate		C/I	C/I
Methylprednisolone sodium succinate	C	C	C
Metoclopramide	I	C	C
Metronidazole	C	C	C
Midazolam	I	I	I
Milrinone	C		
Mitoxantrone	I	C	C
Morphine	C	C/I	I
Nafcillin	C	C	C
Nalbuphine	C	I	I
Netilmicin	C	C	C
Nitroglycerin	C	C	C
Nizatidine	C		
Norepinephrine	C	C	C
Octreotide	C	C	C
Ofloxacin	C	C	C
Ondansetron	C	I	I
Oxacillin	C	C	C
Paclitaxel	C	C	C
Penicillin G potassium	C	C	C
Penicillin G sodium	C	I	I
Pentobarbital	C	I	I
Phenobarbital	C	I	I
Phenytoin	I		I
Phytonadione	C		
Piperacillin	C	C	C
Piperacillin-tazobactam	C	C	C
Prochloperazine edisylate	C	C	C

"Y"-INJECTION SITE MEDICATION COMPATIBILITY WITH PARENTERAL NUTRITION ADMIXTURES[a]

Medication	2-in-1 PN	3-in-1 PN (TNA)	Intravenous lipid emulsions[a]
Promethazine hydrochloride	C/I	C	C
Propofol	C		
Ranitidine	C	C	C
Sargramostin (GM-CSF)	C		
Sodium bicarbonate	I	I	I
Sodium nitroprusside	C	C	C
Tacrolimus	C	C	C
Thiamine			C
Ticarcillin disodium-clavulanate potassium	C	C	C
Tobramycin	C	C	C
Trimethoprim-sulfamethoxazole	C	C	C
Urokinase	C		
Vancomycin	C	C	C
Vecuronium bromide	C		
Vitamin A	C		C
Zidovudine	C	C	

PN = parenteral nutrition; TNA = total nutrient admixture; C = compatible; I = incompatible; C/I = mixed results: preferably do not co-infuse with PN, TNA, or intravenous lipid emulsions.

From: Trissel LA, eds. Handbook on Injectable Drugs. 15th ed. Bethesda: American Society of Health-System Pharmacists;2009.

[a]**Note:** Many Y-site compatibility data with intravenous lipid emulsions were derived from compatibility and stability data with TNA, rather than tested separately with intravenous lipid emulsions.

[b]Human albumin should not be mixed in PN admixtures because of increased infectious risk.

[c]One report showed Y-injection site incompatibility of amikacin at high concentrations of 250 mg/mL with TNA, causing oiling out of the intravenous lipid emulsions, which was not replicated in other similar or lower amikacin concentrations with TNA. Lower amikacin concentration at 5 mg/mL with propofol at the Y-site resulted in a white precipitate, and yellow color formed immediately.

[d]One report showed microscopic globule coalescence when ascorbic acid 500 mg was added to intravenous lipid emulsion solution. Other solution compatibility reports with higher ascorbic acid doses showed physical compatibility for up to 24 hours.

[e]Tested with propofol at Y-site, and caused lipid emulsion to break and oil out.

[f]Y-site incompatibility showed white precipitate formation at cefazolin concentrations of 20 mg/mL with PN admixture, which was not replicated in other similar or higher cefazolin concentrations with PN and TNA.

[g]**Note:** Ceftriaxone should not be used in neonates $\leq$ 28 days old when receiving or expected to receive calcium-containing intravenous products, because of lethal risk for precipitates in lungs and kidneys.

[h]Solution compatibility showed aggregation of oil droplets with intravenous lipid emulsions and cloxacillin.

[i]Heparin incompatibility with TNAs caused flocculation and separation of phases of the intravenous lipid emulsion. This is caused by the negatively charged heparin interacting with positively charged sites of the lipid particles that is facilitated by calcium binding or bridging. However, this is mostly observed at high heparin concentrations.

For more information on intravenous medication compatibility, contact the Drug Information Service (phone 734-936-8200) during work hours, or the 24-hour satellite inpatient Pharmacies (Mott Children's Hospital Pharmacy, phone 734-764-8208; Main Hospital 6th floor Pharmacy, phone 734-936-8251).

APPENDIX L

RECOMMENDED DIETARY ALLOWANCES FOR ENERGY REQUIREMENTS IN PEDIATRICS[1]

	Age (years)	Weight (kg/lb)	Height (cm/in)	Average energy requirements (kcal/kg/day)
Infants	0.0–0.5	6/13	60/24	108
	> 0.5–0.9	9/20	71/28	98
Children	1–3	13/20	90/35	102
	4–6	20/44	112/44	90
	7–10	28/62	132/52	70
Males	11–14	45/99	157/62	55
	15–18	66/145	176/69	45
Females	11–14	46/101	157/62	47
	15–18	55/120	163/64	40

[1] The Recommended Dietary Allowances (RDAs) are intended to provide for individual variations among most normal persons as they live in the United States under usual environmental stresses. Diets should be based on a variety of common foods to provide other nutrients for which human requirements have been less well defined.

From: Food and Nutrition Board, National Academy of Sciences–National Research Council Recommended Dietary Allowances, Revised 1989.

Note: the RDAs have been replaced by the Dietary Reference Intakes (DRIs). For complete and updated listing of DRIs, visit the Institute of Medicine website at: http://www.iom.edu/.

APPENDIX M
Preterm and Transitional Infant Formulas and Human Milk Fortifier

Formula	Enfamil Premature LIPIL 20/24, Low Iron, Iron Fortified®	Similac Special Care 20/24 with Iron®	Similac Neosure 22®	Enfamil Enfacare LIPIL 22®	Enfamil Human Milk Fortifier® (Powder) (per 4-0.025 g pkts)
Description/ Indication	Low birthweight infant	Low birthweight infant	Premature infant transitional	Premature infant transitional	Human breast milk fortifier
Caloric density (Kcal/mL)	0.67/0.8	0.67/0.8	0.74	0.74	12 kcal (4 kcal/pkt)
Protein (g/L) (% total calories)	20/24 (12)	20/24 (12)	21 (11)	19 (11)	1.1 (32)
Source	Non-fat milk, Whey protein concentrate	Non-fat milk, Whey protein concentrate	Non-fat milk, Whey protein concentrate	Non-fat milk, Whey protein concentrate	Milk protein isolate, Whey protein isolate hydrolysate
Fat (g/L) (% total calories)	34/41 (44)	37/44 (47)	41 (49)	36 (47)	1 (63)
Source	MCT (40%), Soy, High-oleic sunflower and/or safflower oils, ARA/DHA (3%)	MCT (50%), Soy, Coconut Oils (0.25% DHA, 0.4% ARA)	MCT (25%), Soy, Coconut oils (0.15% DHA, 0.4% ARA)	MCT (20%), Soy, Coconut, High-oleic vegetable oils, (0.32 DHA)	MCT (70%), Soy oil
Carbohydrate (g/L) (% total calories)	73/90 (44)	70/84 (41)	75 (40)	70 (42)	<0.4
Source	Corn syrup solids, Lactose (60:40)	Corn syrup solids, Lactose (50:50)	Corn syrup solids, Lactose (50:50)		Corn syrup solids, Mineral salts
Water (g/L)	887/880	886	893	811	0.08
Vitamins (/L)					
Vitamin A, IU	8338/10000	8454/10162	3422	3330	950
Vitamin D, IU	1600/1920	1014/1227	522	592	150
Vitamin E, IU	42/50	27/32.5	27	29.6	4.6
Vitamin K, mcg	53/64	81/97	82	59	4.4
Vitamin C, mg	133/160	250/300	112	118	12
Thiamine (B1), mg	1.33/1.6	1.7/2	1.6	1.5	0.15
Riboflavin (B2), mg	2/2.4	4.2/5	1.1	1.5	0.2
Niacin, mg	27/32	33.8/41	14.5	14.8	3
Pyridoxine (B6), mg	1/1.2	1.7/2	0.74	0.74	0.12
Folic acid, mcg	266/320	250/300	186	192	25
Vitamin B12, mcg	1.7/2	3.7/4.5	3	2.2	0.18
Pantothenic acid, mg	8/9.6	12.9/15	6	6.3	0.73
Biotin, mcg	27/32	250/300	67	44	2.7
Choline, mg/L	133/160	68/81	119	178	n/a
Inositol, mg/L	293/352	271/325	260	222	n/a
Carnitine, mg/L	16/19.2	--/48	53	15	n/a
Taurine, mg/L	40/48	--/45	55	44	n/a
Minerals (/L)					
Calcium, mg (mEq)	1100 (55)/1320 (66)	1217/1461 (73)	781 (39)	888 (44)	90
Phosphorus, mg	553/664	676/812	461	488	50
Sodium, mg (mEq)	386 (17)/464 (20)	291/350 (15)	245 (11)	259 11)	16
Potassium, mg (mEq)	653 (17)/784 (20)	872/1050 (27)	1056 (27)	777 (20)	29
Chloride, mg	600 (17)/720 (20)	548/660 (19)	560 (16)	577 (16)	13
Magnesium, mg	60/72	81/98	67	59	1
Iron, mg	3.3 (12)/4 (14.4)*	12.2/14.6	13.4	13.3	1.44
Zinc, mg	10/12	10/12	9	9.3	0.72
Copper, mg	0.8/0.96	1.7/2	0.9	0.9	0.044
Manganese, mg	0.04/0.05	0.08/0.1	0.07	0.1	0.01
Selenium, mcg	19/22	12.2/14.6	17	21	n/a
Iodine, mcg	167/200	41/49	112	155	n/a
Osmolality (mOsm/Kg water)	240/300	235/280	250	250	Adds 35 to breast milk
Renal solute load (mOsm/L)	180/220	188/226	187	181	97
Comments:	*Numbers in parentheses are iron-fortified feeds.				

APPENDIX M (continued)
Milk-Based Infant Formulas

Formula	Enfamil LIPIL/ Lactofree LIPIL®	Enfamil LIPIL 24 cal/oz, Ready to Feed®	Similac Advance®	Carnation Good Start Supreme®
Description/ Indication	Milk-based, full-term infant formula	Milk-based, full-term infant formula	Milk-based, full-term infant formula	Milk-based, full-term infant formula
Caloric density (Kcal/mL)	0.67	0.8	0.67	0.67
Protein (g/L) (% total calories)	14 (8.5)	17 (8.5)	14 (8)	14.7
Source	Non-fat milk, Whey protein concentrate (60:40 whey:casein)/ Milk protein isolate	Reduced minerals whey protein, Non-fat milk	Non-fat milk, Whey protein Concentrate	Partially hydrolyzed reduced minerals whey protein concentrate
Fat (g/L) (% total calories)	35 (48)	42 (48)	36 (49)	
Source	Palm, Soy, Coconut, High-oleic sunflower oils (0.32% DHA, 0.64% ARA)	Palm, Soy, Coconut, High-oleic sunflower oils (contains DHA and ARA)	High-oleic safflower, Coconut, Soy oils (0.15% DHA, 0.4% ARA)	Palm, Soy Coconut, High-oleic safflower or sunflower (0.32% DHA, 0.64% ARA)
Carbohydrate (g/L) (% total calories)	73 (43.5)	87 (43.5)	73 (43)	74.7
Source	Lactose/Corn syrup solids	Lactose	Lactose	Lactose
Water (g/L)	894	872	899	894
Vitamins (/L)				
Vitamin A, IU	2000	2400	2029	2000
Vitamin D, IU	400	480	406	400
Vitamin E, IU	13.3	16	10	13.3
Vitamin K, mcg	53	64	54	53
Vitamin C, mg	80	96	61	60
Thiamine (B1), mg	0.53	0.64	0.67	0.67
Riboflavin (B2), mg	0.93	1.1	1.01	0.93
Niacin, mg	6.7	8	7.1	7
Pyridoxine (B6), mg	0.4	0.5	0.4	0.5
Folic acid, mcg	107	128	101	100
Vitamin B12, mcg	2	2.4	1.7	2.2
Pantothenic acid, mg	3.3	4	3	3
Biotin, mcg	20	24	30	29
Choline, mg/L	160	192	108	160
Inositol, mg/L	40	48	31.7	40
Carnitine, mg/L	13.3	n/a	10	n/a
Taurine, mg/L	40	n/a	40	n/a
Minerals (/L)				
Calcium, mg (mEq)	520(26)/546 (27)	624 (31)	527 (26)	447
Phosphorus, mg	286	344	284	253
Sodium, mg (mEq)	180 (8)/200 (9)	216 (10)	162 (7)	180 (8)
Potassium, mg (mEq)	720 (18)/ 733 (19)	864 (22)	709 (18)	720 (18)
Chloride, mg	420 (12)/446 (13)	504 (14)	439 (12)	434 (12)
Magnesium, mg	53	64	41	47
Iron, mg	12	14.4	12	10
Zinc, mg	6.7	8	5.1	5.3
Copper, mg	0.5	0.6	0.61	0.53
Manganese, mg	0.1	0.12	0.03	0.1
Selenium, mcg	18.6	22.4	12.2	20
Iodine, mcg	67/100	80	41	80
Osmolality (mOsm/Kg water)	300	360	300	250
Renal solute load (mOsm/L)	128	153	126	n/a

168

APPENDIX M (continued)
Soy-Based and Protein Hydrolysate Infant Formulas

Formula	Prosobee 20[®]	Isomil Advance 20[®]	Nutramigen[®]	Pregestimil 20/24[®]	Alimentum[®]
Description/ Indication	Soy protein	Soy protein	Protein hydrolysate	Protein hydrolysate with MCT	Protein hydrolysate with MCT
Caloric density (Kcal/mL)	0.67	0.67	0.67	0.67/0.8	0.67
Protein (g/L) (% total calories)	16.7 (10)	16.5 (10)	19 (11)	19/23 (11)	19 (11)
Source	Soy protein isolate, L- methionine, L-carnitine	Soy protein isolate, L-methionine, L-carnitine	Casein hydrolysate, L-cystine, tyrosine, L-tryptophan, L-carnitine	Casein hydrolysate, L-cystine, L-tyrosine, L-tryptophan, L-carnitine	Casein hydrolysate, L-cystine, L-tyrosine, L-tryptophan
Fat (g/L) (% total calories)	35 (48)	35 (49)	37 (48)	38/45 (48)	38 (48)
Source	Palm, Soy, Coconut, Sunflower oils (0.32% DHA, 0.64% ARA)	High-oleic Safflower, Coconut, Soy oils	Palm, Coconut, Soy, Sunflower oils (0.32% DHA, 0.64% ARA)	MCT (55%), Corn, Soy, Sunflower oils (0.3% DHA, 0.6% ARA)	MCT (33%), Safflower, Soy oils
Carbohydrate (g/L) (% total calories)	71 (42)	69 (41)	68 (41)	69/83 (41)	69 (41)
Source	Corn syrup solids	Corn syrup solids, Sucrose (80:20)	Corn syrup solids, Modified corn starch	Corn syrup solids, Modified corn starch, Dextrose	Sugar, modified tapioca starch (70:30)
Water (g/L)	887	899	887		899
Vitamins (/L)					
Vitamin A, IU	2000	2029	2000	2535/3040	2029
Vitamin D, IU	400	405	334	334/400	304
Vitamin E, IU	13.3	10	13.3	27/32	20.3
Vitamin K, mcg	53	74	53	80/96	101
Vitamin C, mg	80	61	80	80/96	61
Thiamine (B1), mg	0.54	0.4	0.53	0.54/0.64	0.4
Riboflavin (B2), mg	0.6	0.6	0.6	0.6/0.7	0.61
Niacin, mg	6.7	9.1	6.7	6.7/6.7	9.1
Pyridoxine (B6), mg	0.4	0.4	0.4	0.4/0.5	0.41
Folic acid, mcg	107	101	107	107/128	101
Vitamin B12, mcg	2	3	2	2/2.4	3
Pantothenic acid, mg	3.3	5	3.3	3.3/4	5.1
Biotin, mcg	20	30.4	20	20/24	30.4
Choline, mg/L	160	81	160	160/192	81
Inositol, mg/L	40	33.8	113	113/136	33.8
Carnitine, mg/L	13.3	10	13.3	13.3/16	n/a
Taurine, mg/L	40	51	40	40/48	n/a
Minerals (/L)					
Calcium, mg (mEq)	700 (35)	710 (35)	627 (31)	627 (31)/752 (38)	710 (35.4)
Phosphorus, mg	460	507	347	347/416	507
Sodium, mg (mEq)	240 (10.3)	297 (12.8)	313 (13.6)	313 (13.6)/376(16)	298 (12.9)
Potassium, mg (mEq)	800 (21)	730 (19)	733 (19)	733 (19)/880 (23)	798 (20.3)
Chloride, mg	533 (15)	419 (11.5)	574 (16.4)	574 (16)/688 (20)	541 (15.5)
Magnesium, mg	73	51	73	73/88	50.7
Iron, mg	12	12.2	12	12/14.4	12.2
Zinc, mg	8	5	6.7	6.7/8	5.1
Copper, mg	0.5	0.51	0.5	0.5/0.6	0.51
Manganese, mg	0.17	0.17	0.17	0.17/0.2	0.54
Selenium, mcg	18.6	12.2	18.9	18.9/22.4	12.2
Iodine, mcg	100	101	100	100/120	101
Osmolality (mOsm/Kg water)	170	200	320	320/340	370
Renal solute load (mOsm/L)	156	154	168	169/200	171

Formula	Portagen 20®	Similac PM 60/40®	EleCare®	Neocate®
Description/ Indication	MCT-rich for chylous ascites, Chylothorax	Lower mineral content, milk-based	Elemental hypoallergenic	Elemental hypoallergenic with ARA and DHA
Caloric density (Kcal/mL)	0.67	0.67	0.67	0.67
Protein (g/L) (% total calories)	24 (14)	15 (9)	20.6 (15)	20.9 (12)
Source	Sodium caseinate	Whey protein concentrate, sodium caseinate	Free amino acids	Free amino acids
Fat (g/L) (% total calories)	32 (40)	38 (50)	32.7 (42)	30 (41)
Source	MCT (87%), Corn oil	High-oleic Safflower, Soy and Coconut oils	MCT (33%), Soy oil, High-oleic Safflower oil	MCT (5%), Soy, Coconut, High-oleic Safflower oils
Carbohydrate (g/L) (% total calories)	78 (46)	69 (41)	72.4 (43)	79 (47)
Source	Corn syrup solids, Sugar	Lactose	Corn syrup solids	Corn syrup solids
Water (g/L)	910	899	895	875
Vitamins (/L)				
Vitamin A, IU	5320	2029	1846	2765
Vitamin D, IU	532	406	284	405
Vitamin E, IU	21	10.1	14.2	7.7
Vitamin K, mcg	106	54	40.5	59
Vitamin C, mg	55	61	61	63
Thiamine (B1), mg	1.06	0.68	1.4	0.6
Riboflavin (B2), mg	1.27	1	0.7	0.9
Niacin, mg	14.1	7.1	11.4	10.4
Pyridoxine (B6), mg	1.41	0.4	0.57	0.83
Folic acid, mcg	106	101	199	69
Vitamin B12, mcg	4.2	1.7	2.8	1.7
Pantothenic acid, mg	7	3	2.8	4.2
Biotin, mcg	53	30.4	28	21
Choline, mg/L	88	81	64	89
Inositol, mg/L	32	162	34	158
Carnitine, mg/L	12.7	n/a	48.3	n/a
Taurine, mg/L	40	n/a	92.4	n/a
Minerals (/L)				
Calcium, mg (mEq)	634 (32)	379 (19)	781 (39)	838 (42)
Phosphorus, mg	475	189	568	629
Sodium, mg (mEq)	373 (16)	162 (7)	305 (13.3)	252 (11)
Potassium, mg (mEq)	848 (22)	541 (13.8)	1015 (26)	1048 (26.8)
Chloride, mg	590 (17)	399 (11.3)	405 (11.4)	523 (14.9)
Magnesium, mg	141	40.6	57	84
Iron, mg	12.7	4.7	9.9	12.5
Zinc, mg	6.3	5.1	5.7	11.2
Copper, mg	1.06	0.6	0.7	0.84
Manganese, mg	0.85	0.03	0.57	0.6
Selenium, mcg	n/a	12.2	15.6	25.2
Chromium, mcg	n/a	n/a	15.6	24
Molybdenum, mcg	n/a	n/a	17	32
Iodine, mcg	49	41	57	104
Osmolality (mOsm/Kg water)	230	280	350	375
Renal solute load (mOsm/L)	200	124	187	n/a

Formula	Nutren Jr./Nutren Jr. with fiber[®**]	Resource Just For Kids 1.5/ JFK 1.5 w/ fiber***[®]	Peptamen Junior[®]	Neocate One +[®]	Vivonex Pediatric[®]
Description/ Indication	Oral or enteral formula	Concentrated oral or enteral	Protein hydrolysate	Elemental hypoallergenic	Elemental hypoallergenic
Caloric density (Kcal/mL)	1	1.5	1	1	0.8
Protein (g/L) (% total calories)	30 (12)	42 (11)	30 (12)	25 (10)	24 (12)
Source	Milk protein, Whey protein concentrate	Sodium/calcium caseinates, whey protein concentrate	Enzymatically hydrolyzed whey protein	100% free amino acids	100% free amino acids
Fat (g/L) (% total calories)	50 (44)	75 (45)	38.4 (33)	35 (32)	24 (25)
Source	MCT (21%), Canola oil	MCT (11%), Soy, High-oleic Sunflower oil	MCT (60%), Canola, Soy oils	MCT (35%), Canola, High-oleic Safflower oils	MCT (69%), Soybean oil
Carbohydrate (g/L) (% total calories)	110 (44)	165 (44)	138 (55)	146 (58)	130 (63)
Source	Maltodextrin, Sucrose 6 g fiber (2.2 g soluble, 3.8 g insoluble)	Maltodextrin, Sugar 9 g, fiber from partially hydrolyzed guar gum, soy fiber	Maltodextrin	Corn syrup solids	Maltodextrin Modified corn starch
Water (g/L)	852	720 (712 w/ fiber)	848	850	893
Vitamins (/L)					
Vitamin A, IU	4068	3000	4064	1170	2500
Vitamin D, IU	560	460	560	310	500
Vitamin E, IU	28	23	28	8.2	30
Vitamin K, mcg	60	40	30	15	40
Vitamin C, mg	100	100	100	31	100
Thiamine (B1), mg	2.4	1.2	2.4	0.55	1.5
Riboflavin (B2), mg	2	1.5	2	0.65	1.8
Niacin, mg	20	19	20	9	20
Pyridoxine (B6), mg	2.4	1.6	2.4	0.8	2
Folic acid, mcg	400	370	400	60	200
Vitamin B12, mcg	6	2.4	6	0.7	3
Pantothenic acid, mg	10	10	10	2.4	5
Biotin, mcg	300	150	300	20	100
Choline, mg/L	300	400	300	183	200
Inositol, mg/L	80	120	80	18	60
Carnitine, mg/L	40	26	40	31.7	25
Taurine, mg/L	80	130	80	50	80
Minerals (/L)					
Calcium, mg (mEq)	1000 (50)	1300 (65)	1000 (50)	620 (31)	970 (48.5)
Phosphorus, mg	800	990	800	620	800
Sodium, mg (mEq)	460 (20)	690 (30)	460 (21)	200 (9)	400 (17)
Potassium, mg (mEq)	1320 (34)	1300 (33)	1320 (33.8)	930 (23.8)	1200 (31)
Chloride, mg	1080 (29)	750 (21)	1080 (30)	350 (10)	1000 (28)
Magnesium, mg	200	200	200	90	200
Iron, mg	14	14	14	7.7	10
Zinc, mg	15.2	12	15.2	7.7	12
Copper, mg	1	1.1	1	1	1.2
Manganese, mg	1.6	2.3	1.6	1	2
Selenium, mcg	30	34	30	15	30
Chromium, mcg	30	69	24.4	30	45
Molybdenum, mcg	60	58	48	35	75
Iodine, mcg	120	140	120	60	120
Osmolality (mOsm/Kg water)	350	390 (405 with fiber)	260 380 (vanilla)	610	360
Renal solute load (mOsm/L)	256	n/a	255	n/a	n/a

INDEX

A

M

N

SELECTED BIBLIOGRAPHY

ALUMINUM

Canada TW. Aluminum exposure through parenteral nutrition formulations: mathematical versus clinical relevance [published correction appears in Am J Health Syst Pharm 2005;62:679]. Am J Health Syst Pharm 2005;62:315-8.

Driscoll M, Driscoll DF. Calculating aluminum content in total parenteral nutrition admixtures. Am J Health Syst Pharm 2005;62:312-5.

CARNITINE

Crill CM, Helms RA. The use of carnitine in pediatric nutrition. Nutr Clin Pract 2007;22:204-13.

Crill CM, Christensen ML, Storm MC, et al. Relative bioavailability of carnitine supplementation in premature neonates. JPEN J Parenter Enteral Nutr 2006;30:421-5.

CHOLESTASIS ASSOCIATED WITH PARENTERAL NUTRITION

Btaiche IF, Khalidi N. Parenteral nutrition-associated liver dysfunction in children. Pharmacotherapy 2002;22:188-211.

CRITICAL ILLNESS AND NUTRITION SUPPORT

Elke G, Schädler D, Engel C, et al. German Competence Network Sepsis (SepNet). Current practice in nutritional support and its association with mortality in septic patients; results from a national, prospective, multicenter study. Crit Care Med 2008;36:1762-7.

McClave SA, DeMeo MT, DeLegge MH, et al. North American Summit on Aspiration in the Critically Ill Patient: consensus statement. JPEN J Parenter Enteral Nutr 2002;26(suppl):S80-S85.

Heyland DK, Dhaliwal R, Drover JW, et al. Canadian clinical practice guidelines for nutrition support in mechanically ventilated, critically ill, adult patients. JPEN J Parenter Enteral Nutr 2003;27:355-73.

DEXTROSE INFUSION IN PEDIATRIC PATIENTS

Farrag HM, Cowett RM. Glucose homeostasis in the micropremie. Clin Perinatol 2000; 27:1-22.

Bendorf K, Friesen CA, Roberts CC. Glucose response to discontinuation of parenteral nutrition in patients less than 3 years of age. JPEN J Parenter Enteral Nutr 1996;20:120-2.

Cowett RM, Oh W, Pollak A, et al. Glucose disposal of low birth infants: steady state hyperglycemia produced by constant intravenous glucose infusion. Pediatrics 1979;63:389-96.

ENERGY EXPENDITURE AND METABOLISM

McClave SA, Snider HL. Use of indirect calorimetry in clinical nutrition. Nutr Clin Pract 1992; 7:207-21.

Harris JA, Benedict FG. A biometric study of basal metabolism in man. Carnegie Institution of Washington, Washington; 1919.

ENTERAL NUTRITION

Btaiche IF, Chan LN, Pleva M, Kraft MD. Critical illness, gastrointestinal complications, and medication therapy during enteral feeding in critically ill adult patients. Nutr Clin Pract 2010;25:32-49.

Lewis SJ, Andersen HK, Thomas S. Early enteral nutrition within 24 h of intestinal surgery versus later commencement of feeding: a systematic review and meta-analysis. J Gastrointest Surg 2009;13:569-75.

Koretz RL. Do data support nutrition support? Part II. Enteral artificial nutrition. J Am Diet Assoc 2007;107:1374-80.

Koretz RL, Avenell A, Lipman TO, et al. Does enteral nutrition affect clinical outcome? A systematic review of the randomized trials. Am J Gastroenterol 2007;102:412-29.

McClave SA, Lukan JK, Stefater JA, et al. Poor validity of residual volumes as a marker for risk of aspiration in critically ill patients. Crit Care Med 2005;33:324-30.

Lewis SJ, Egger M, Sylvester PA, et al. Early enteral feeding versus "nil by mouth" after gastrointestinal surgery: systematic review and meta-analysis of controlled trials. BMJ 2001;323:1–5.

Mentec H, Dupont H, Bocchetti M, et al. Upper digestive intolerance during enteral nutrition in critically ill patients: frequency, risk factors, and complications. Crit Care Med 2001;29:1955-61.

Marik PE, Zaloga GP. Early enteral nutrition in acutely ill patients: a systematic review. Crit Care Med 2001;29:2264-70.

ENTERAL VERSUS PARENTERAL NUTRITION

Woodcock NP, Zeigler D, Palmer MD, et al. Enteral versus parenteral nutrition: A pragmatic study. Nutrition 2001;17:11-12.

ESSENTIAL FATTY ACIDS

Lee EJ, Simmer K, Gibson RA. Essential fatty acids in parenterally fed preterm infants. J Paediatr Health 1993;29:51-5.

Sardesai VM. The essential fatty acids. Nutr Clin Pract 1992;7:179-86.

FLUIDS AND ELECTROLYTES

Dickerson RN, Henry NY, Miller PL, et al. Low serum total calcium concentration as a marker of low serum ionized calcium concentration in critically ill patients receiving specialized nutrition support. Nutr Clin Pract 2007;22:323-8.

Dickerson RN, Morgan LM, Croce MA, et al. Dose-dependent characteristics of intravenous calcium therapy for hypocalcemic, critically ill, trauma patients receiving specialized nutritional support. Nutrition 2007;23:9-15.

Kraft MD, Btaiche IF, Sacks GS, et al. Treatment of electrolyte disorders in adult patients in the intensive care unit. Am J Health-Syst Pharm 2005;62:1663-82.

Dickerson RN, Gervasio JM, Sherman JJ, et al. A comparison of renal phosphorus regulation in thermally-injured and multiple-trauma patients receiving specialized nutrition support. JPEN J Parent Enteral Nutr 2001;25:152-9.

Clark CL, Sacks GS, Dickerson RN, et al. Treatment of hypophosphatemia in patients receiving specialized nutrition support using a graduated dosing scheme: results from a prospective clinical trial. Crit Care Med 1995;23:1504-11.

GUIDELINES AND SAFE PRACTICES OF NUTRITION SUPPORT

McClave SA, Martindale RG, Vanek VW, et al. A.S.P.E.N. Board of Directors; the American College of Critical Care Medicine. Guidelines for the provision and assessment of nutrition support therapy in the adult critically ill patient: Society of Critical Care Medicine (SCCM) and American Society for Parenteral and Enteral Nutrition (A.S.P.E.N.). JPEN J Parenter Enteral Nutr 2009;33:277-316.

Mehta NM, Compher C. A.S.P.E.N. Board of Directors. A.S.P.E.N. Clinical guidelines: nutrition support of the critically ill child. JPEN J Parenter Enteral Nutr 2009;33:260-76.

Bankhead R, Boullata J, Brantley S, et al. A.S.P.E.N. Board of Directors. Enteral nutrition practice recommendations. JPEN J Parenter Enteral Nutr 2009;33:122-67.

Rollins C, Durfee SM, Holcombe BJ, et al; ASPEN Task Force for Revision of Nutrition Support Pharmacist Standards. Standards of practice for nutrition support pharmacists. Nutr Clin Pract 2008;23:189-94.

Kreymann KG, Berger MM, Deutz NE, et al; DGEM (German Society for Nutritional Medicine); Ebner C, Hartl W, Heymann C, et al; ESPEN (European Society for Parenteral and Enteral Nutrition). ESPEN guidelines on enteral nutrition: intensive care. Clin Nutr 2006;25:210-23.

Mirtallo J, Canada T, Johnson D, et al; Task Force for the Revision of Safe Practices for Parenteral Nutrition. Safe practices for parenteral nutrition [published correction appears in JPEN J Parenter Enteral Nutr 2006;30:177]. JPEN J Parenter Enteral Nutr 2004;28(6):S39-S70.

The American Society for Parenteral and Enteral Nutrition, Board of Directors and the Clinical Guidelines Task Force. Guidelines for the use of parenteral and enteral nutrition in adult and pediatric patients. JPEN J Parenter Enteral Nutr 2002;26:1S-138S.

American Gastroenterological Association, Clinical Practice and Practice Economics Committee.AGA technical review on parenteral nutrition. Gastroenterology 2001;121:970-1001.

The American Society for Parenteral and Enteral Nutrition, National Advisory Group on Standards and Practice Guidelines for Parenteral Nutrition. Safe practices for parenteral nutrition formulations. JPEN J Parenter Enteral Nutr 1998;22:49-66.

Heyland DK, MacDonald S, Keefe L, et al. Total parenteral nutrition in the critically ill patient. A Meta-analysis. JAMA 1998; 280:2013-9.

FDA Safety Alert: Hazards of precipitation associated with parenteral nutrition. Am J Hosp Pharm 1994;51:1427-8.

HOME NUTRITION SUPPORT

Dickerson RN, Brown RO. Parenteral and enteral nutrition in the home and chronic-care settings. Am J Manag Care 1998;4:445-55.

HYPERGLYCEMIA AND HYPOGLYCEMIA

Finfer S, Chittock DR, Su SY, et al. The NICE-SUGAR study investigators. Intensive versus conventional glucose control in critically ill patients. N Engl J Med 2009;360:1283-97.

Dickerson RN, Swiggart CE, Morgan LM, et al. Safety and efficacy of a graduated intravenous insulin infusion protocol in critically ill trauma patients receiving specialized nutrition support. Nutrition 2008;24:536-45.

Krinsley JS, Grover A. Severe hypoglycemia in critically ill patients: risk factors and outcomes. Crit Care Med. 2007;35:2262-7.

Butler SO, Btaiche IF, Alaniz C. Relationship between hyperglycemia and infection in critically ill patients. Pharmacotherapy 2005;25:963-76.

Van Den Berghe G, Woutres P, Weekers F, et al. Intensive insulin therapy in critically ill patients. N Engl J Med 2001; 345:1359-67.

Rosmarin DK, Wardlaw GM, Mirtallo J. Hyperglycemia associated with high, continuous infusion rates of total parenteral nutrition dextrose. Nutr Clin Pract 1996;11:151-6.

HYPOCALORIC FEEDING

Dickerson RN. Hypocaloric feeding of obese patients in the intensive care unit. Curr Opin Clin Nutr Metab Care 2005;8:189-96.

IMMUNONUTRITION

Marik PE, Zaloga GP. Immunonutrition in critically ill patients: a systematic review and analysis of the literature. Intensive Care Med 2008; Jul 15.

Kudsk KA, Moore FA. Proceedings from summit on immune-enhancing enteral therapy. JPEN J Parenter Enteral Nutr 2001;25(2 suppl):1S-63S.

INSULIN AND HYPERGLYCEMIA IN LOW BIRTH WEIGHT INFANTS

Kanarek KS, Santeiro ML, Malone JI. Continuous infusion of insulin in hyperglycemic low-birth weight infants receiving parenteral nutrition with and without lipids. JPEN J Parenter Enteral Nutr 1991;15:417-20.

INTRAVENOUS LIPID EMULSIONS

Bach AC, Férézou J, Frey A. Phospholipid-rich particles in commercial parenteral fat emulsions. An overview. Prog Lipid Res 1996;35:133-53.

Tashiro T, Mashima Y, Yamamori H, et al. Increased lipoprotein X causes hyperlipidemia during intravenous administration of 10% fat emulsion in man. JPEN J Parenter Enteral Nutr 1991;15:546-50.

Carpentier YA. Intravascular metabolism of fat emulsions. Clin Nutr 1989; 8:115-25.

INTRAVENOUS LIPID EMULSIONS IN LOW-BIRTH-WEIGHT INFANTS

Wells DH, Ferlauto JJ, Forbes DJ, et al. Lipid tolerance in the very low-birth-weight infant on intravenous and enteral feedings. JPEN J Parenter Enteral Nutr 1989;13:263-7.

American Academy of Pediatrics, Committee on Nutrition: nutritional needs of low-birth-weight infants. Pediatrics 1985; 75:976-86.

LIVER DISEASE

Cabré E, Gassull MA. Nutrition in liver disease. Curr Opin Clin Nutr Metab Care 2005;8:545-51.

Btaiche IF. Branched-chain amino acids in patients with hepatic encephalopathy. Nutr Clin Pract 2003;18:97-100.

METABOLIC COMPLICATIONS ASSOCIATED WITH PARENTERAL NUTRITION

Btaiche IF, Khalidi N. Metabolic complications of parenteral nutrition in adults, parts 1 & 2. Am J Health-Syst Pharm 2004;61:1938-49; 2050-9.

NEONATES

Valentine CJ, Puthoff TD. Enhancing parenteral nutrition therapy for the neonate. Nutr Clin Pract 2007;22:183-93.

Ziegler EE, Thureen PJ, Carlson SJ. Aggressive nutrition of the very low-birth-weight infant. Clin Perinatol 2002;29:225-44.

Kalhan S, Bier D, Yaffe S, et al. Protein/amino acid metabolism and nutrition in very low-birth-weight infants. J Perinatol 2001;21:320-3.

Newell SJ. Enteral feeding of the micropremie. Clin Perinatol 2000; 27:221-34.

Thureen PJ, Anderson AH, Baron KA, et al. Protein balance in the first week of life in ventilated neonates receiving parenteral nutrition. Am J Clin Nutr 1998;38:1128-35.

NITROGEN BALANCE

Konstantinides FN, Konstantinides NN, Li JC, et al. Urinary urea nitrogen: too insensitive for calculating nitrogen balance studies in surgical clinical nutrition. JPEN J Parenter Enteral Nutr 1991; 15:189-93.

Loder PB, Kee AJ, Horsburgh R, et al. Validity of urinary urea nitrogen as a measure of total urinary nitrogen in adult patients requiring parenteral nutrition. Crit Care Med 1989;17:309-12.

NUTRITION AND METABOLISM IN PRETERM INFANTS

Greer FR. Vitamin metabolism and requirements in the micropremie. Clin Perinatol 2000; 27:95-118.

Leitch CA, Denne SC. Energy expenditure in the extremely low-birth-weight infant. Clin Perinatol 2000; 27:181-95.

Hay WW, Lucas A, Heird WC, et al. Workshop summary: nutrition of the extremely low-birth-weight infant. Pediatrics 1999;104:1360-8.

NUTRITIONAL MARKERS

Marshall WJ. Nutritional assessment: its role in the provision of nutritional support. J Clin Pathol 2008;61:1083-8.

Carlson DE, Cioffi WG, Mason AD, et al. Evaluation of serum visceral protein levels as indicators of nitrogen balance in thermally injured patients. JPEN J Parenter Enteral Nutr 1991;15:440-4.

Boosalis MG, Ott L, Levine AS, et al. Relationship of visceral proteins to nutritional status in chronic and acute stress. Crit Care Med 1989;17:741-7.

PANCREATITIS

Curtis CS, Kudsk KA. Nutrition support in pancreatitis. Surg Clin North Am 2007;87:1403-15.

McClave SA, Chang WK, Dhaliwal R, et al. Nutrition support in acute pancreatitis: a systematic review of the literature. JPEN J Parenter Enteral Nutr 2006;30:143-56.

Marik PE, Zaloga GP. Meta-analysis of parenteral nutrition versus enteral nutrition in patients with acute pancreatitis. BMJ 2004;328:1407-12.

PARENTERAL NUTRITION FOR ADULTS

Koretz RL. Parenteral nutrition and urban legends. Curr Opin Gastroenterol 2008;24:210-4.

Koretz RL. Do data support nutrition support? Part I: intravenous nutrition. J Am Diet Assoc 2007;107:988-96.

PERIOPERATIVE PARENTERAL NUTRITION

The Veterans Affairs Total Parenteral Nutrition Cooperative Study Group. Perioperative total parenteral nutrition in surgical patients. N Engl J Med 1991;325:525-32.

PERMESSIVE UNDERFEEDING

Rubinson L, Diette GB, Song X, et al. Low-caloric intake is associated with Nosocomial bloodstream infections in patients in the medical intensive-care unit. Crit Care Med 2004;32:350-7.

Jeejeebhoy KN. Permissive underfeeding of the critically ill patient. Nutr Clin Pract 2004;19:477-80.

PHARMACEUTICAL ISSUES WITH PARENTERAL NUTRITION

Bertch KE, McKinnon BT. Pharmaceutical issues for parenteral nutrition solutions. In: Christensen ML, McKinnon BT, eds. Nutrition Support Pharmacy. Selected cases for self-study. Silver Spring, MD: American Society for Parenteral and Enteral Nutrition; 1995;7:1-16.

PREGNANCY AND NUTRITION

The HAPO Study Cooperative Research Group. Hyperglycemia and Adverse Pregnancy Outcomes. N Engl J Med 2008;358:1991-2002.

Institute of Medicine. Nutrition during pregnancy. Washington, DC: National Academy Press; 1990.

Kirby DF, Fiorenza V, Craig RM. Intravenous nutritional support during pregnancy. JPEN J Parenter Enteral Nutr 1988;72-80.

REFEEDING SYNDROME

Kraft MD, Btaiche IF, Sacks GS, et al. Treatment of electrolyte disorders in adult patients in the intensive-care unit. Am J Health-Syst Pharm 2005;62:1663-82.

RENAL FAILURE

Btaiche IF, Mohammad R, Alaniz C, et al. Amino acid requirements in critically ill, acute renal-failure patients treated in continuous renal replacement therapy. Pharmacotherapy 2008;28:600-13.

Churchwell MD, Pasko DA, Btaiche IF, et al. Trace-element removal during in vitro and in vivo continuous haemodialysis. Nephrol Dial Transplant 2007;22:2970-7.

Wooley JA, Btaiche IF, Good KL. Metabolic and nutritional aspects of acute renal failure in critically ill patients requiring continuous renal replacement therapy. Nutr Clin Pract 2005;20:176-91.

SHORT BOWEL SYNDROME

Cole CR, Hansen NI, Higgins RD, et al. Very low-birth-weight preterm infants with surgical short bowel syndrome: incidence, morbidity, and mortality, and growth outcomes at 18 to 22 months. Pediatrics 2008;122:e573-82.

O'Keefe SJ, Buchman AL, Fishbein TM, et al. Short bowel syndrome and intestinal failure: consensus definitions and overview. Clin Gastroenterol Hepatol 2006;4:6-10.

Buchman AL, Scolapio J, Fryer J. AGA technical review on short bowel syndrome and intestinal transplantation. Gastroenterology 2003;124:1111-34.

TOTAL NUTRIENT ADMIXTURES

Driscoll DF. Total nutrient admixtures: Theory and practice. Nutr Clin Pract 1995;10:114–119.

TRACE ELEMENTS

Angstwurm MW, Gaertner R. Practicalities of selenium supplementation in critically ill patients. Curr Opin Clin Nutr Metab Care 2006;9:233-8.

Dickerson RN. Manganese intoxication and parenteral nutrition. Nutrition 2001;17:689-93.

Braunschweig CL, Sowers M, Kovacevich DS, et al. Parenteral zinc supplementation in adult humans during the acute phase response increases the febrile response. J Nutr 1997;127:70-4.

Baker SS, Lerman RH, Krey SH, et al. Selenium deficiency with total parenteral nutrition: reversal of biochemical and functional abnormalities by selenium supplementation: a case report. Am J Clin Nutr 1983;38:769-74.

VITAMINS

Dickerson RN, Garmon WM, Kuhl DA, et al. Vitamin K-independent warfarin resistance after concurrent administration of warfarin and continuous enteral nutrition. Pharmacotherapy 2008;28:308-13.

Helphingstine CJ, Bistrian BR. New food and drug administration requirements for inclusion of vitamin K in adult parenteral multivitamins. JPEN J Parenter Enteral Nutr 2003;27:220-4.

Snow CF. Laboratory diagnoses of vitamin B12 and folate deficiency: a guide for the primary care physician. Arch Intern Med 1999;159:1289-98.

NOTES

NOTES